Measuring and Monitoring Cov
Interventions in Women, Children and
in Low and Middle Income Countries

C000115049

Edited by

Agbessi Amouzou (Institute for International Programs, Department of International Health, Johns Hopkins Bloomberg School of Public Health, Baltimore, Maryland, USA)

Jennifer Harris Requejo (Data and Analytics Section, Division of Research and Policy, UNICEF, New York, New York, USA)

Liliana Carvajal (Data and Analytics Section, Division of Research and Policy, UNICEF, New York, New York, USA)

Doris Chou (Department of Reproductive Health and Research, World Health Organization, Geneva, Switzerland)

Hannah H. Leslie (Department of Global Health, Harvard TH Chan School of Public Health, Boston, Massachusetts, USA)

Safia S. Jiwani (Institute for International Programs, Department of International Health, Johns Hopkins Bloomberg School of Public Health, Baltimore, Maryland, USA)

William Weiss (Department of International Health, Johns Hopkins Bloomberg School of Public Health, Baltimore, Maryland, USA)

Published in the United Kingdom by Inishmore Laser Scientific Publishing Ltd.

Inishmore Laser Scientific Publishing Ltd.
Caledonian Exchange, 19a Canning St, Edinburgh,
United Kingdom, EH3 8HE

Logo: Qubrik Ltd, Edinburgh, UK

Printed in Croatia by LaserPLUS, Ltd.

ISBN-13: 978-1-9999564-8-6

Measuring and Monitoring Coverage of Health Interventions in Women, Children and Adolescents in Low and Middle Income Countries

Edited by

Agbessi Amouzou (Institute for International Programs, Department of International Health, Johns Hopkins Bloomberg School of Public Health, Baltimore, Maryland, USA)

Jennifer Harris Requejo (Data and Analytics Section, Division of Research and Policy, UNICEF, New York, New York, USA)

Liliana Carvajal (Data and Analytics Section, Division of Research and Policy, UNICEF, New York, New York, USA)

Doris Chou (Department of Reproductive Health and Research, World Health Organization, Geneva, Switzerland)

Hannah H. Leslie (Department of Global Health, Harvard TH Chan School of Public Health, Boston, Massachusetts, USA)

Safia S. Jiwani (Institute for International Programs, Department of International Health, Johns Hopkins Bloomberg School of Public Health, Baltimore, Maryland, USA)

William Weiss (Department of International Health, Johns Hopkins Bloomberg School of Public Health, Baltimore, Maryland, USA)

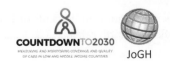

COUNTDOWN TO 2030

MEASURING AND MONITORING COVERAGE AND QUALITY OF CARE IN LOW AND MIDDLE INCOME COUNTRIES

JoGH

Contents

Naima T Joseph, Ellen Piwoz, Dennis Lee, Address Malata, Hannah H Leslie; on behalf of the Countdown Coverage Technical Working Group

SECTION 3

DETERMINANTS OF COVERAGE

Althea Andrus, Robert Cohen, Liliana Carvajal, Shams El Arifeen, William Weiss

Dr. Agbessi Amouzou is a demographer and currently an Associate Professor in the Department of International Health at the Johns Hopkins Bloomberg School of Public Health, in Baltimore, USA.

His interests are on approaches for measuring and monitoring child mortality and coverage of high impact maternal, newborn and child health (MNCH) programs in low and middle-income countries (LMIC), and the evaluation of the effectiveness of large scale MNCH programs in LMIC. He currently leads the development and implementation of a countrywide sample registration system for mortality and cause of death measurement in Mozambique, and the MNCH coverage analysis as part of the Countdown to 2030 initiative. For two and half years, he led the MNCH coverage data analysis for global and country monitoring at UNICEF Headquarters in New York, and currently co-chairs the Countdown to 2030 Coverage Technical Working Group.

Dr. Jennifer Harris Requejo is a Senior Advisor, Statistics and Monitoring, in the Data and Analytics Unit at UNICEF Headquarters, New York. She currently leads the Health and HIV team which includes the content areas of HIV, immunization, and maternal, newborn, child and adolescent health. She previously served as the Technical Deputy Director for Countdown to 2030 and was a Senior Technical Officer at the Partnership for Maternal, Newborn & Child Health hosted by the World Health Organization. She also was an Associate Scientist in the Department of International Health at the Johns Hopkins Bloomberg School of Public Health, Baltimore. She currently co-chairs the Countdown to 2030 Coverage Technical Working Group and oversees the development and production of the Countdown to 2030 national country profiles.

Liliana Carvajal, MA, MSc Epi, works as Statistics and Monitoring Specialist at the Data and Analytics Section of the Division of Data Analysis Planning and Monitoring at UNICEF. She is an epidemiologist with over 10 years of experience in global health. Liliana currently coordinates the data and analysis work in the areas of maternal, newborn, child and adolescent health. Over the past two years, Liliana has been leading the measurement work on mental health among adolescents at the population level. Liliana was recently on assignment in Senegal contributing to the coordination and M&E work of the multi-country Child Friendly Communities/ Real Time Monitoring project. She has been working over the years on global, regional and national M&E priorities including data analysis across the continuum of care for maternal, newborn, child and adolescents' health as well as on methodological development of data collection methods.

Prior to her current role at UNICEF, Liliana worked as analyst for the Human Development Report Office of UNDP. She holds a Master's degree in International Political Economy and Development, from Fordham University in New York and a Master of Science in Epidemiology from the London School of Hygiene and Tropical Medicine in London.

Dr. Doris Chou has been based in Geneva, Switzerland since 2009 as a Medical Officer in the Department of Sexual and Reproductive Health and Research of the World Health Organization. Until 2019, Doris led the monitoring and evaluation portfolio of the Department, focusing on maternal mortality and tracking targets as they relate to ending preventable maternal mortality and the achievement of the SDGs. Her areas of focus included global maternal mortality estimation, causes of maternal death classification, and estimation.

In her current role, she coordinates the portfolio related to norms and standards for maternal health, including the living guideline process. Recent work focuses on shining a light on the burden of non-communicable diseases in maternal health and making the case for a better understanding of the problem so that it is both recognised and effectively addressed by countries and health systems.

Dr Chou is an obstetrician gynaecologist, sub-specializing in maternal-fetal medicine. Prior to joining the WHO, she was an Assistant Professor in the Division of Maternal Fetal Medicine at the University of Pennsylvania in Philadelphia, PA. During her tenure there, her clinical interests were diagnostic ultrasound and she undertook research related to viral placental infection.

Dr. Hannah H. Leslie, PhD MPH, Research Scientist, Harvard TH Chan School of Public Health. Dr. Leslie is an epidemiologist and global health researcher with particular expertise in health system measurement and quality of care. She leads studies on the efficient assessment of health care quality in low-resource settings and on implications of quality for population health behaviors and outcomes. This work includes design of tools to capture health system and population perspectives on health services as well as quantitative analysis of large existing datasets. One of her areas of focus is effective coverage measurement: developing better methods for capturing the impact of health systems on population health and applying these methods to complex data from low- and middle-income countries alike. Dr. Leslie was the Research Lead on Measurement for the *Lancet Global Health* Commission on High Quality Health Systems in the Sustainable Development Goal Era, she serves on the Countdown to 2030 Technical Working Group on Coverage, and she contributed to the WHO Think Tank Series on Effective Coverage Measurement.

Safia S. Jiwani, MSPH, received her training in nutrition, public health and epidemiology. She is passionate about maternal newborn and child health in low- and middle-income countries and the double burden of malnutrition. Her research interests are centered around improving the measurement of MNCH coverage indicators and quality of care in LMICs, and measuring health inequalities. Safia has over 5 years of experience in global health with the International Medical Corps, the Pan American Health Organization, and CARE US. She currently works as a Research Associate in the Department of International Health at the Johns Hopkins Bloomberg School of Public Health, where she is a member of the Countdown to 2030 Coverage Technical Working Group, and coordinates a nationwide mortality surveillance system in Mozambique.

Dr. William Weiss, DrPH, MA, Senior Associate with the Department of International Health, Johns Hopkins Bloomberg School of Public Health. Dr. Weiss's career focus is in health information systems, assessment, monitoring and evaluation of public health and humanitarian assistance programs in low- and middle-income countries. At Johns Hopkins, he is an instructor in the following international health courses: Health Information Systems, Design and Implementation of Global Digital Health interventions, and Applying Household Surveys to PHC Programs. He is also a lecturer in several other courses including Measurement Methods in Emergencies and Public Health Surveillance. At USAID, he is a senior advisor on metrics- and digital health-related activities to the Office of Maternal and Child Health and Nutrition. His DrPH degree is in international health at Johns Hopkins Bloomberg School of Public Health. His MA degree in International Affairs is from The George Washington University with a focus in International Development. A cross-section of his practice experience includes the following activities: monitoring the quality and outcomes of clinical care supported by numerous government and NGO health programs in Africa, Asia and Latin America (malaria and pneumonia case management, HIV/AIDS anti-retroviral therapy or HAART); principal investigator for both cohort studies and randomized trials related to HAART, leadership and management, and mental health interventions; assessing immunization coverage following vaccination campaigns; qualitative study of child health practices and beliefs and problems of persons affected by torture or trauma; participatory planning and action activities with IDP communities in Northern Uganda and Northern Sudan; and, household surveys of maternal and child health practices in Africa and Asia.

PREFACE

Countdown to 2030's global health experts completed new analyses on how women, children and adolescents are being reached with high impact life saving interventions in low and middle-income countries. This series presents indicators and key determinants of service coverage and discusses future research on strategies to improve RMNCAH&N services and reduce inequalities.

Countdown to 2030 is a consortium of measurement experts from academia and UN organizations, tracking the progress of life saving interventions for women, children and adolescent health and nutrition. We provide the most recent data and analysis on equity and coverage of RMNCAH&N services to support leaders to make evidence-based decisions to improve health outcomes.

Acknowledgment

The series was produced on behalf of Countdown to 2030's Coverage Technical Working Group: Agbessi Amouzou (co-chair), Jennifer Requejo (co-chair), Shams El Arifeen, Robert Black, Ties Boerma, Liliana Carvajal, Doris Chou, Chika Hayashi, Sennen Hounton, Safia Jiwani, Youssouf Keita, Margaret Kruk, Hannah Leslie, Mengjia Liang, Honorati Masanja, Purnima Menon, Allisyn Moran, Lois Park, Lara Vaz, Shelley Walton, William Weiss.

We would like to acknowledge Shelley Walton (Johns Hopkins University) for her coordination support, Brittany Furgal (Johns Hopkins University) for her logistical support and Rie Tai (Johns Hopkins University) for her communications and graphics support. We are grateful to the Bill & Melinda Gates Foundation for funding Countdown to 2030 for Women's Children's and Adolescents' Health through US Fund for UNICEF.

Overview

The importance of improving intervention coverage measurement for ensuring all women, children and adolescents are reached with the health care services they need

Jennifer Requejo[1], Agbessi Amouzou[2]

[1] Division of Data, Analysis, Planning and Monitoring, United Nations Children's Fund, New York, New York, USA

[2] Department of International Health, Johns Hopkins University, Baltimore, Maryland, USA

The United Nations General Assembly adopted the Sustainable Development Goal Framework (SDGs) in September 2015 with a set of 17 goals and 169 targets to be achieved by 2030 [1]. The Global Strategy for Women's, Children's and Adolescents' Health (2016-2030), in support of Every Women Every Child (EWEC GS) [2], was launched shortly afterwards to translate the broad SDG agenda into concrete guidance on how to ensure every woman, child and adolescent can realize their right to the highest-attainable standard of health. Regular monitoring of progress towards the SDG and EWEC GS goals is essential for determining where efforts need to be accelerated, where lessons can be learned and scaled up, and to hold us all to account for our roles in making universal health coverage a reality. Embedded in the EWEC GS is a monitoring framework that includes a set of indicators which cover the dimensions of survive, thrive and transform. The Countdown to 2030 indicator list complements and expands upon the EWEC GS indicator set by focusing on intervention coverage and equity in coverage. The Countdown indicators are organized into two main categories: Those that capture information about effective interventions for improving maternal, newborn, and child survival and for which comparable, high quality data are available; and those for which further measurement work is needed so that standards can be put into place for data collection, reporting and interpretation.

In addition to reporting on the first category of indicators through the Countdown country profiles and associated analyses [3], a central remit of the Countdown to 2030 Coverage Technical Working Group is to improve the measurement of this second category of core indicators on women's, children's and adolescents' health. The aim of this measurement work is to increase the availability of timely data for assessing progress and for helping countries modify existing programs and develop new programs to increase coverage of high-quality interventions and ultimately improve health outcomes. This supplement presents a diverse set of secondary analyses undertaken by the Countdown to 2030 Coverage Technical Working Group. It focuses on intervention coverage and effective coverage measurement in the 81 highest maternal and child mortality burden countries. The collection of articles in the supplement build off previous analyses of intervention coverage conducted and published under the Child Health and Epidemiology Reference Group (CHERG) (http://collections.plos.org/measuring-coverage-in-mnch) and Countdown to 2015, the predecessor of Countdown to 2030, (http://www.tandfonline.com/toc/zgha20/8/s5). Each article explores measurement challenges or levels, trends and correlates of specific indicators related to women's, children's and adolescents' health and nutrition, identifies strategies to increase the coverage of the interventions captured through these indicators, and suggests ways forward for addressing remaining data and research gaps.

The article by Amouzou et al [4], for example, investigates the discordance in intervention coverage for postnatal care for mothers and postnatal care for babies, finding that a large proportion of this variance is related to the current approach for measuring postnatal care which does not adequately distinguish between intrapartum and postnatal care. Suggestions are made for addressing the challenge of capturing the timing of intrapartum care compared to a first postnatal care visit. The paper authored by Jiwani et al [5] explores indicators available on the number, timing and content of antenatal care in 54 countries with a Demographic Health Survey or Multiple Indicator Cluster Survey conducted since 2012. Her analysis shows that antenatal care initiation in these countries is a key factor in the total number of visits received and is directly related to key social determinants such as women's education level and living in rural areas. The paper from Andrus et al. [6] focusses on predictors of coverage of treatment for diarrheal diseases, which remain a leading cause of child deaths, particularly in low-and-middle income countries. Her paper finds that community-based interventions are critical for increasing coverage of oral rehydration solution as are strategies for reducing out of pocket expenditures for treatment services for childhood illnesses. The article led by Trivedi and colleagues [7] assesses country progress towards the elimination of mother to child transmission of syphilis and HIV with a focus on syphilis. The findings indicate that countries need additional support and options for affordable and integrated testing platforms to expand syphilis screening during antenatal care visits. Treatment services for women testing positive for syphilis also need to be scaled up to reduce congenital syphilis cases. Using household survey and available health facility data from Malawi, Joseph and colleagues [8] point out that although many women are accessing antenatal care, they are not receiving recommended nutrition interventions crucial for their health and the health of their babies. This study highlights the importance of linking available data sources to improve our understanding of the content of maternal health services. Sauer and colleagues tackle the challenge of estimating the variance of measures of effective coverage that combine data from multiple sources such as household and quality of care surveys. They examine the performance of three methods – the exact, delta, and parametric bootstrap methods – and formulate recommendations for the appropriate method to use based the data at hand [9].

In sum, this short collection of articles helps advance our understanding of progress in reaching all women, children and adolescents with essential health interventions, and demonstrates how the use of innovative methodological approaches to linking available data sources can shed light on gaps in the quality of care that must be addressed. Work on improving measurement and monitoring of intervention coverage needs to be supported throughout the SDG era so that we can best help countries shape programs and policies that will result in universal health coverage and lead them on the pathway to achieving the SDGs.

Acknowledgments: We would like to thank all of the authors involved in the supplement and Brittany Furgal and Shelley Walton for their logistical and administrative support.

Funding; This paper was supported by a grant from the Bill & Melinda Gates Foundation for the Countdown to 2030 initiative.

Authorship contributions: *JR and AA conceptualized and wrote the paper.*

Competing interests: *The authors completed the ICMJE Unified Competing Interest form (available upon request from the corresponding author), and declare no conflicts of interest.*

Reference

1 World Health Organization. Sustainable Development Goal Framework. 2015. Available: https://sustainabledevelopment.un.org/post2015/transformingourworld. Accessed: 20 February 2020.

2 World Health Organization. The Global Strategy for Women's Children's and Adolescents'. Health. 2015. Available: https://www.who.int/life-course/partners/global-strategy/global-strategy-2016-2030/en/. Accessed February 20, 2020.

3 Countdown to 2030. Country profiles. Available: http://countdown2030.org/country-profiles. 2020. Accessed:20 February, 2020.

4 Amouzou A, Hazel E, Vaz L. Discordance in postnatal care between mother and newborn: Measurement artifact or missed opportunity. J Glob Health. 2020;10:010505. doi:10.7189/jogh.10.010505

5   Jiwani SS, Amouzou A, Carvajal L, Chou D, Keita Y, Moran A, et al. Timing and number of antenatal care contacts in low and middle-income countries: Analysis in the Countdown to 2030 priority countries. J Glob Health. 2020;10:010502. doi:10.7189/jogh.10.010502

6   Andrus A, Cohen R, Carvajal-Aguirre L, El Arifeen S, Weiss W. Strong community-based health systems and national governance predict improvement in coverage of oral rehydration solution (ORS): a multilevel longitudinal model. J Glob Health. 2020;10:010503. doi:10.7189/jogh.10.010503

7   Trivedi S, Taylor M, Kamb ML, Chou D. Improving syphilis screening and treatment in ANC to prevent congenital syphilis. J Glob Health. 2020;10:010504. doi:10.7189/jogh.10.010504

8   Joseph NT, Piwoz E, Lee D, Malata A, Leslie H. Examining coverage, content, and impact of maternal nutrition interventions: the case for quality-adjusted coverage measurement. J Glob Health. 2020;10:010501. Medline:32082545 doi:10.7189/jogh.10.010501

9   Sauer SM, Pullum T, Wang W, Mallick L, Leslie H. Variance estimation for effective coverage measures: A simulation study. J Glob Health. 2020;10:010506.doi:10.7189/jogh.10.010506

Section 1

Coverage data and measurement

Discordance in postnatal care between mothers and newborns: Measurement artifact or missed opportunity?

Agbessi Amouzou[1], Elizabeth Hazel[1], Lara Vaz[2], Sanni Yaya[3], Allisyn Moran[4]

---

[1] Department of International Health, Johns Hopkins Bloomberg School of Public Health, Baltimore, Maryland, USA

[2] Save the Children, Washington, D.C., USA

[3] School of International Development and Global Studies, University of Ottawa, Ottawa, Ontario, Canada

[4] World Health Organization, Geneva, Switzerland

Background Postnatal care (PNC) for mothers and newborns is essential to monitor risks of morbidity and adverse conditions following delivery. Current estimates of the coverage of PNC show substantial discordance between mothers and newborns. We investigate the sources of this discordance in Demographic and Health Surveys (DHS).

Methods We used DHS data from 48 countries collected since 2011, spanning phases 6 and 7 of the survey program with 32 and 16 surveys, respectively, analyzed. We assessed the distribution of the reported timing of PNC and conducted a sensitivity analysis that excludes/includes PNC reported within 0-1 hour or PNC in the day 2. Agreement in PNC reporting considered four groups: (1) Concordance, neither mother nor newborn received PNC; (2) Concordance, mother and newborn pair received PNC; (3) Discordance, mother received PNC and newborn did not; of (4) Discordance, mother did not receive PNC but the newborn did. We carried out logistic regressions to understand correlates of PNC discordance. All analyses distinguished phase 6 surveys from phase 7.

Results We found substantial differences in the PNC coverage estimated between phase 6 and phase 7 surveys. The phase 7 PNC questions for newborns were improved to increase the understanding of the questions by respondent which probably led to reducing the large PNC gap between mothers and newborns observed in phase 6 surveys. With phase 6 surveys, PNC coverage for mother was estimated on average at 62% compared to only 31% for newborns. No such gap was observed for phase 7 surveys, where for both mothers and newborns, the PNC coverage estimate was similar, at 56%. For both phases, over half of the reported PNC for mothers and newborns occurred during 0-1 hour following delivery, leading to substantial overestimation of PNC coverage, due to confusion between intrapartum care and PNC. There were 37% discordant cases between mother and newborn, largely in favor of the mother in phase 6 surveys, compared to 16% in phase 7 surveys. In phase 6 surveys, discordant PNC cases were observed largely among facility deliveries vs non-facility deliveries (44% compared to 19%).

Conclusions Current estimates of coverage of PNC from DHS phase 6 surveys appears to include substantial level of measurement noises that could explain substantial part of the mother-newborn discordance in PNC. The PNC estimates appear to capture a substantial number of intrapartum care. Current measurement approaches warrant further validation to ensure accurate monitoring of the PNC programs.

Postnatal care for mothers and newborns is a critical package of interventions to monitor the health status of mothers and newborns during the six weeks following delivery. It has been shown to be effective in reducing neonatal mortality [1-3]. The 2013 WHO guidelines prescribe integrated postnatal care for the both the mother and the newborn, with the first health check occurring within the first 24 hours after birth. Three additional health checks for the mother and newborn are recommended successively on day three, between day seven and fourteen, and six weeks after birth. For facility deliveries, care must be provided in the facility for at least 24 hours [4]. The recommended content for newborn postnatal care includes an assessment of the newborn for any abnormal signs, exclusive breastfeeding, and cord care. For the mother, a complete assessment, complemented with iron and folic acid supplementation, counseling and psychosocial support are recommended. Postnatal care is distinct from immediate newborn care which includes resuscitation, thermal care and breastfeeding initiation. For the mother, providers check for signs of hemorrhage and infection during the 24 hours and continue monitoring health throughout the postnatal period and is distinct from intrapartum care [5].

Measuring the coverage of postnatal care contacts in household surveys has been challenging; Moran et al discussed extensively the measurement challenges of postnatal care for both the woman and the newborn [6]. To date, only a postnatal care contact indicator has been defined at global level and adopted by countries. The global indicator defines postnatal care contact as health check received within two days of delivery. The two largest household survey programs in low- and middle-income countries, the Demographic and Health Surveys (DHS) and the Multiple Indicator Cluster Surveys (MICS), have developed approaches to measure this indicator. Although efforts have been made by the two survey programs to harmonize their approaches, they continue to implement slightly different algorithms for measurement, which makes comparability difficult [7].

Furthermore, the assessment of postnatal care contacts indicates substantial level of discrepancy in the report of care received by the mother and the newborn. The Countdown to 2030, which monitors coverage of effective interventions in 81 countries in LMIC, reported median postnatal care for mothers at 59% compared to 42% for babies for the period 2012-2016 [8]. Such a result is surprising given the recommendation for integrated postnatal care for both mother and newborn. The discrepancy may be indicative of the quality of postnatal care service provision. It can also originate from misreporting from mothers based on their understanding of the questions, their recall of postnatal services received, and whether mother and newborn have been separated at some point following the delivery, leading the mother to be unaware of any care provided to the newborn, including the possibility that only one of the dyad is actually receiving PNC.

The discordance in PNC for mother and newborn has not been studied in the literature. This paper assesses this discordance in low and middle-income countries with available recent DHS surveys. More specifically, we quantify the gap in coverage of PNC for mothers and newborns, the level of discordance and concordance in reporting of PNC between mothers and newborn within individual dyads. We assess the reported timing of PNC and carry out sensitivity analysis to understand whether there is possible confusion between intrapartum care and postnatal care, the possibility of differential recall by respondent during the household survey, and the effect it has on coverage estimates. Finally, we analyze socio-demographic, economic and service provision factors associated with the likelihood of discordance in reported receipt of PNC.

DATA AND METHODS

We used available data from Demographic and Health Surveys (DHS) carried out since 2011. DHS is a nationally representative sample survey carried out generally about every five years in most low and middle-income countries. The survey interviews head of households, all women aged 15-49 and men aged 15-59 (or 15-64 in some cases). Women's interviews include information on their complete birth history. For women who had a birth in the past five years, additional health-related questions, including maternal and newborn care questions, are posed. We retained most recent surveys which included questions measuring postnatal care of both woman and newborn and restricted the analysis to births in the two years preceding the survey. Data were downloaded from the DHS website (dhsprogram.com) as of 4th April 2019. A total of 48 countries are included in the analysis, representing 280 651 births in the two years preceding the surveys. This includes 32 surveys from phase 6 (accounting for 223 500 births) and 16 surveys from phase 7 (accounting for 57 151 births). Table S1 in the **Online Supplementary Document** includes the list of countries included in the analysis.

The PNC questions in DHS

The DHS program revises its questionnaire according to phases of five years. Data since 2011 span phases 6 (DHS6) and 7 (DHS7). The questionnaire module for newborn PNC was expanded starting in phase 7. **Figure 1** and **Figure 2** show the questions asked to elicit PNC information in the respective survey phases. There were differences in the wording and structure of the questions between the two phases. For mothers, the set of questions were similar between the two phases regardless of place of birth. For newborns, DHS7 distinguished between facility vs non-facility births and asked a separate set of questions for each; DHS6 on the other hand, had a single question regardless of place of birth. Furthermore, a two-month window was included in the newborn PNC questions in DHS6; in DHS7, this window was referenced only for non-facility births and facility births for whom the mother reported that no health check was performed on the newborn before discharge. Questionnaire differences between DHS6 and DHS7 are a potential source of measurement differences in the PNC coverage estimates.

The PNC indicator

While the WHO guidelines recommend several PNC contacts with specific timing, for measurement and monitoring, the global community has focused mainly on the first contact. The global PNC contact indicator is defined as PNC intervention received within 48 hours of delivery, regardless of the place of delivery [5]. The PNC indicator captures contact with a health provider and the timing of the contact. For both mothers and newborns, we calculated the global indicator, restricting to deliveries in the past two years preceding the survey to reduce potential effects of recall.

Statistical analysis

We carried out descriptive analysis of PNC indicators and a multilevel logit regression of PNC discordance. Given the 48 hours window following the birth that is used to define the global PNC indicator, a major constraint affecting the indicator is the ability to distinguish intrapartum and essential newborn care provided immediately following delivery to mothers and newborns from actual postnatal care. To understand this possible overlap, we first analyze the timing of the reported first PNC contact to capture its distribution. We then carried out sensitivity analyses of the global PNC indicator by including/excluding the first PNC reported to have occurred within 0 or 1 hour. Similarly, there is usually a reporting confusion between day 0 and day 1 making it possible that day 2 is counted as part of the 48 hours following delivery. We therefore also compared

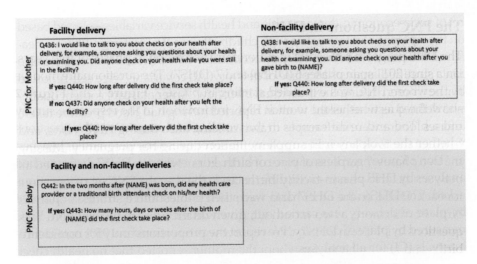

Figure 1. *DHS 6 design for postnatal care questions for mothers and newborns.*

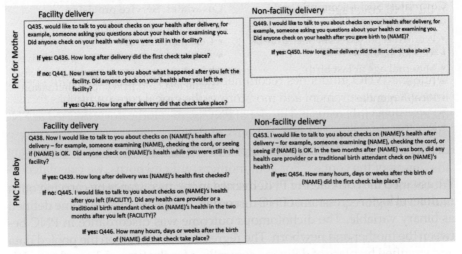

Figure 2. *DHS 7 design for postnatal care questions for mothers and newborns.*

the PNC contact indicator, including/excluding day 2. We carried out the analyses by country and also for the pooled country data sets.

To analyze the PNC contact discordance between mother and newborn we distinguished four categories: (1) negative concordance with neither mother nor newborn received PNC; (2) positive concordance when both mother and newborn pair received PNC; (3) "mother-favored" discordance based on mother received PNC and her newborn did not; and (4) "newborn-favored" discordance based on mother did not receive PNC but the newborn did. We analyzed the association between the type of concordance/discordance and a set of socio-economic, demographic and health service variables, selected based on their potential relationship with childbirth (see **Box 1**). Given PNC is measured differently whether delivery occurred in a health facility or not, we also ran a stratified analysis by place of delivery. All covariates were self-reported by the women during the individual interview. Antenatal care content quality was defined as whether the woman reported having had blood pressure taken, and a blood and urine sample drawn at least once during ANC visits, and whether she took any iron supplementation during her pregnancy. Missing or "Don't Know" responses were considered as "No". We further stratified all analyses by DHS phases given differences in the way the PNC questions were asked. The DHS6 and DHS7 data were then pooled and a stratified analysis by place of delivery was carried out, given differences in the way PNC was measured by place of delivery. We report the proportions and 95% confidence intervals (CI) for all analyses.

Box 1. *Covariates included in the analysis.*

Covariates: Socio-economic and demographic variables	Covariates: Service provision
• Women reported level of education • Marital status • Maternal age at last birth • Parity • Wealth quintile • Proceeding birth interval • Whether the child is still alive • Months since last birth	• Place of delivery (facility vs other) • Cesarean delivery • ANC content quality (having received blood pressure assessment, blood and urine test, and iron supplementation during the index pregnancy)

We assessed the correlates of PNC discordance/concordance by carrying out a multilevel logit regression of PNC discordance/concordance outcome defined as binary variable. The dichotomous outcome was discordance in PNC between the mother and newborn. The regressions were run on the pooled data and stratified by place of delivery, controlling for the type of discordance. We used Stata 14 with for all analysis (Stata Corp, College Station, TX, USA). For reporting proportions and 95% confidence intervals, we used the *svy* command in Stata, taking into account sampling weights, enumeration area clustering and stratified design. To account for differential sample size in the pooled data, the descriptive analysis was weighted by the inverse of the proportion of births in the past two years preceding the survey in each country.

Ethical clearance

All data used are publicly available. Ethical clearance was the responsibility of the institutions that collected the data.

RESULTS

Reported timing of PNC

Figure 3 shows the timing of reported PNC contact for mothers and newborns by phase of the DHS. The distribution of PNC timing for mothers and for newborn appears similar across mothers and newborn and within each survey phase. The report of first PNC contact decreases rapidly beyond 1 hour; another peak is observed on day 1 followed with a decline in subsequent days.

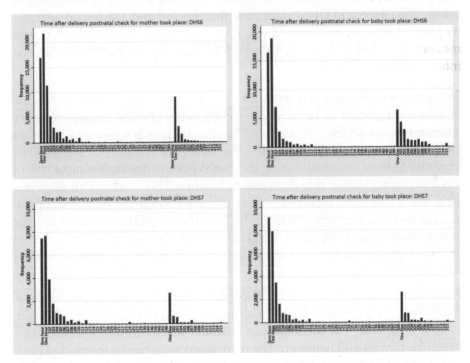

Figure 3. *Timing of reported first prenatal care (PNC) contact after delivery for mothers and newborn, by phase of Demographic and Health Survey (DHS).*

Sensitivity analysis of PNC coverage to reported timing

To capture the effects of the report of timing of the PNC contact on the overall PNC coverage indicator, **Figure 4** shows results of sensitivity analysis comparing the global PNC indicator (red square) to other variants computed separately for DHS 6 and 7 phases. These variants are: (1) PNC within 2 days, with any PNC reported to have occurred during 0 or 1 hour considered as no PNC (blue diamond); (2) PNC within two days with report of 0-1 hour timing excluded from the analysis (purple triangle); and (3) PNC within two days,

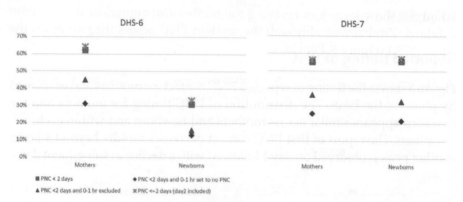

Figure 4. *Sensitivity of postnatal care (PNC) indicators: comparison of PNC indicators for mothers and newborns, excluding/including 0-1 hours and/or day 2.*

including reported day 2 (green star). Further pooled and country specific results are included in Table S2, S3 and S4 in the **Online Supplementary Document**. For DHS6, coverage of PNC for mothers is substantially higher than that of babies, while for DHS7, the levels are similar. For DHS6, PNC reported to have occurred during the first 0-1 hour constitute almost half of PNC occurring within two days among women: PNC within two days was 62%, but when those reported to have occurred within 0-1 hour are considered as no PNC, the indicator drops to 31%. The drop is from 31% to 13% for newborn. Thus, for both mothers and babies, half of the report of PNC appears to have occurred within 0-1 hour of delivery. When PNC within 0-1 hour is excluded from the analysis, the drop reduces substantially for mothers only (from 62% to 45%). Similar results are observed for DHS7, although the drop between PNC within two days and PNC within two days with 0-1 set to no PNC was slightly more pronounced for babies (from 56% to 22%) than for mothers (55% to 26%).

Gap between the Coverage of PNC for mothers and PNC for newborns

There is a substantial gap in PNC coverage between mothers and babies in favor of mothers, especially for surveys of DHS6 (**Figure 5**). The overall gap in the median PNC across the 48 surveys is as large as 30 percentage points in favor of the mother (62% for mothers and 32% for babies), originating mostly from the gap in DHS 6 surveys, for which the median gap is as wide as 42 percentage points (65% for mothers and 23% for babies). For these surveys, the gap is over 50 percentage points (pp) in Gambia (71 pp), Egypt (71 pp), Guatemala (65 pp), and Ghana (59 pp) (**Figure 5**, Panel B). For DHS7, a few countries show large gap favoring the mother (Myanmar) or the newborn (Malawi, Zimbabwe), although the median PNC across the surveys is the same (55%) (**Figure 5**, Panel C).

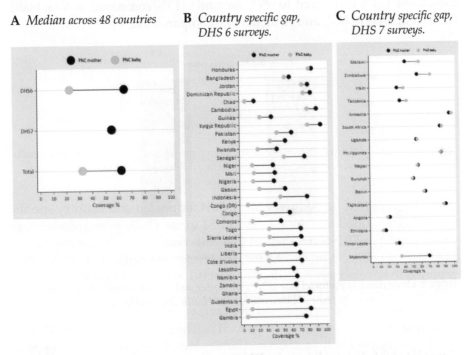

A *Median across 48 countries*   **B** *Country specific gap, DHS 6 surveys.*   **C** *Country specific gap, DHS 7 surveys.*

Figure 5. *Gap in the coverage of postnatal care (PNC) for mothers and newborns.* **Panel A.** *Median gap across 48 countries.* **Panel B.** *Country specific gap, Demographic and Health Survey (DHS) 6 surveys.* **Panel C.** *Country specific gap, DHS 7 surveys.*

Level of discordance in PNC for mother and the newborn

Figure 6 and **Figure 7** present the level of discordance/concordance between PNC mother and PNC newborn respectively in the pooled data across surveys stratified by DHS phase and by specific countries. Consistent with previous results, there is a substantially higher level of discordance in PNC between mother and babies from DHS 6 surveys than from DHS 7. Across the DHS 6 survey, discordance is observed in 37% of cases, and largely skewed in favor of the mother: 34% of mother received PNC while their babies did not, while the opposite occurred in only 3% of the cases. The total level of discordance across DHS 7 surveys is 16%, equally distributed between mothers and babies. Large variation in the level of discordance is observed across countries, ranging from 73% in Egypt and Gambia to 8% in Honduras for DHS 6 surveys, and from 37% in Myanmar to 7% in Armenia and Tajikistan. There are a few countries, especially with DHS 7, in which babies are favored in PNC than mothers. These includes Malawi (21% of mothers reported no PNC for themselves while the babies received one, compared 5% for the opposite), Zimbabwe (21% compared to 6%), Tanzania (13% compared to 6%), Haiti (12% compared to 4%), and Armenia (5% compared to 2%).

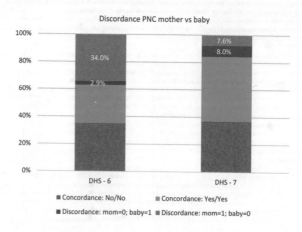

Figure 6. *Discordance in postnatal care (PNC) for mother and newborn, pooled data across surveys by phase of Demographic and Health Survey (DHS).*

Correlates of discordance in PNC

Table 1 shows the percentage of mothers/babies by type of discordance/concordance according to socio-demographic characteristics and health service provision indicators. The table also shows 95% confidence intervals allowing comparison of the percentage across categories of the covariates. As shown above, level of discordance is largely in favor of the mother than the newborn and this is reflected across all characteristics considered. Thus, we focus on this type of discordance. A key set of results is related to service provision variables such the place of birth, receipt of antenatal care routine interventions, and delivery with cesarean section. Mothers who delivered in a health facility were largely more likely to report discordant PNC between themselves and their newborn than those who delivered outside a health facility who were more likely to report negative concordance. Among mothers who delivered in a health facility, 30% (95% CI = 29.7-30.6) had "mother-favored" discordance PNC compared to only 13% (95% CI = 12.3-13.3) among those who delivered outside facilities. This result appears to come mainly from DHS 6 surveys, where 44% of facilities deliveries had discordance compared to 19% among non-facility deliveries. Among DHS7, no such gap in discordance was observed

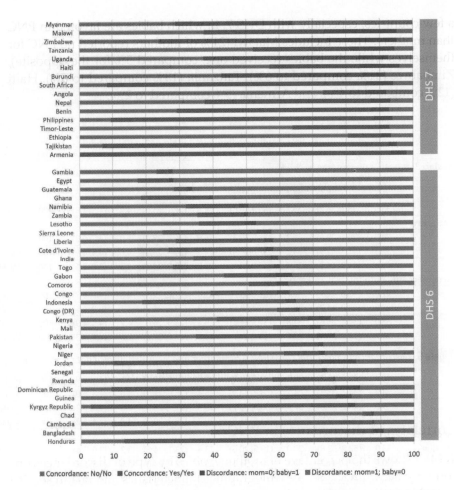

Figure 7. *Discordance in postnatal care (PNC) for mother and newborn, by country and according to the survey phase.*

between facility and non-facility deliveries (8% vs 7%, respectively) (Table S5 in the **Online Supplementary Document**). A related finding is when the mother reported receiving routine ANC interventions such as blood pressure assessment, blood and urine test, iron supplementation. Mothers who reported having received all these interventions during ANC were more likely to report higher level of mother-favored discordance (30% (95% CI = 29.8-30.9) vs 19% (95% CI = 18.9-19.7)). Furthermore, mothers who had caesarian section were more likely to report higher level of mother-favored (36% (95% CI = 35.0-37.1) vs 24% (95% CI = 23.2-24.0)).

There were also varying associations based on socio-demographic characteristics. While there is no difference in the level of discordance according to

Table 1. *Percentage of mother/newborn by type of discordance/concordance with postnatal care (PNC) by socio-demographic and service provision characteristics*

Characteristics	% Concordance No/No		% Concordance Yes/Yes		Discordance, Mom-Yes Baby-No		Discordance, Mom-No Baby-Yes		Total (%)	N
	%	95% CI	%	95% CI	%	95% CI	%	95% CI		
Age at last birth (years), category:										
<20	37.9	(37.0, 38.8)	31.5	(30.6,32.3)	25.2	(24.4, 26.0)	5.4	(5.1, 5.8)	100	41,712
20-34	34.4	(33.9, 34.8)	36.1	(35.6,36.5)	25.0	(24.6, 25.4)	4.5	(4.3, 4.7)	100	202,047
35+	39.4	(38.5, 40.3)	31.0	(30.1,32.0)	25.3	(24.5, 26.1)	4.3	(4.0, 4.7)	100	36,892
Months since last birth, category (age of child):										
<6	35.9	(35.3, 36.6)	34.2	(33.5,34.9)	25.5	(24.9, 26.2)	4.4	(4.1, 4.6)	100	71,107
6-11	35.1	(34.4, 35.7)	34.6	(34.0,35.3)	25.6	(25.0, 26.2)	4.7	(4.4, 5.0)	100	73,971
12-23	35.6	(35.1, 36.2)	35.1	(34.5,35.6)	24.6	(24.1, 25.0)	4.7	(4.5, 4.9)	100	135,573
Parity, category:										
1	29.0	(28.4, 29.6)	39.2	(38.5,39.8)	26.9	(26.3, 27.4)	5.0	(4.7, 5.3)	100	84,300
2-3	32.3	(31.7, 32.9)	38.2	(37.6,38.9)	24.8	(24.3, 25.4)	4.6	(4.4, 4.9)	100	106,353
4+	45.6	(44.9, 46.2)	26.4	(25.9,27.0)	23.7	(23.2, 24.3)	4.3	(4.0, 4.5)	100	89,998
Months of preceding birth interval, category:										
<24	41.0	(40.0, 41.9)	32.7	(31.8,33.7)	22.0	(21.2, 22.8)	4.3	(4.0, 4.7)	100	34,669
24-35	43.5	(42.8, 44.3)	28.1	(27.4,28.8)	24.3	(23.6, 24.9)	4.1	(3.9, 4.4)	100	61,023
36+	35.0	(34.4, 35.6)	34.8	(34.3,35.4)	25.4	(24.9, 26.0)	4.7	(4.5, 4.9)	100	107,457
First birth	27.7	(27.1, 28.3)	40.7	(40.0,41.4)	26.6	(26.0, 27.2)	5.0	(4.7, 5.3)	100	77,502
Wealth quintile:										
Poorest	47.5	(46.7, 48.3)	27.9	(27.2,28.7)	20.2	(19.6, 20.8)	4.4	(4.1, 4.7)	100	63,327
Poorer	40.4	(39.6, 41.2)	32.3	(31.5,33.1)	22.8	(22.1, 23.4)	4.6	(4.3, 4.9)	100	60,113
Middle	34.9	(34.1, 35.7)	34.1	(33.2, 34.9)	26.4	(25.6, 27.1)	4.6	(4.3, 5.0)	100	57,153
Richer	29.0	(28.2, 29.8)	37.7	(36.8, 38.7)	28.5	(27.7, 29.3)	4.8	(4.5, 5.2)	100	54,048
Richest	21.4	(20.6, 22.2)	44.6	(43.5, 45.8)	29.2	(28.3, 30.2)	4.8	(4.4, 5.2)	100	46,009
Highest educational level										
No education	53.0	(52.2, 53.8)	20.0	(19.5, 20.6)	23.8	(23.1, 24.5)	3.2	(3.0, 3.4)	100	76,899
Primary	40.6	(39.9, 41.2)	30.4	(29.8, 31.1)	23.5	(22.9, 24.0)	5.5	(5.3, 5.8)	100	82,506
Secondary +	21.1	(20.6, 21.6)	47.0	(46.3, 47.6)	27.0	(26.5, 27.6)	4.9	(4.7, 5.2)	100	121,247
Current marital status:										
Never in union	30.0	(28.8, 31.2)	33.6	(32.2, 35.0)	30.9	(29.6, 32.3)	5.5	(4.9, 6.1)	100	20,106
Married/living with partner	36.0	(35.5, 36.4)	34.8	(34.4, 35.3)	24.7	(24.4, 25.1)	4.5	(4.3, 4.6)	100	246,817
Other	36.2	(34.7, 37.7)	35.0	(33.5, 36.6)	22.7	(21.4, 24.1)	6.0	(5.3, 6.9)	100	13,728
Facility delivery:										
No	72.3	(71.6, 73.0)	11.1	(10.6, 11.5)	12.8	(12.3, 13.3)	3.8	(3.6, 4.1)	100	81,991
Yes	20.4	(20.0, 20.8)	44.5	(44.0, 45.0)	30.2	(29.7,30.6)	5.0	(4.8, 5.1)	100	198,660
Last birth was with caesarean section:										
No	38.7	(38.2, 39.1)	32.9	(32.5, 33.4)	23.6	(23.2, 24.0)	4.8	(4.7, 5.0)	100	247,316
Yes	12.6	(11.9, 13.4)	48.1	(46.9, 49.3)	36.1	(35.0, 37.1)	3.2	(2.8, 3.7)	100	33,335
ANC: Blood pressure taken + Blood sample + Iron + Urine sample:										
No	47.2	(46.6,47.8)	28.9	(28.3, 29.4)	19.3	(18.9, 19.7)	4.6	(4.4, 4.8)	100	133,913
Yes	24.9	(24.5,25.4)	40.1	(39.5, 40.7)	30.4	(29.8, 30.9)	4.6	(4.4, 4.8)	100	146,738
Child is alive:										
No	43.7	(41.9,45.4)	24.1	(22.6, 25.7)	27.2	(25.7, 28.8)	5.0	(4.2, 6.1)	100	9,656
Yes	35.3	(34.9,35.7)	35.1	(34.7, 35.5)	25.0	(24.6, 25.4)	4.6	(4.5, 4.8)	100	270,995

CI – confidence interval, ANC – antenatal care

the age of the woman at the last birth or the child age at the time of survey, mothers with first birth and those with lower parity were more likely to report discordance than other women. Among mothers with parity one, 27% had mother-favored discordance compared to 25% among mothers with parity 2 or 3, and 24% among those with parity 4 or more. Birth interval is also associated with level of discordance, with shorter birth interval corresponding to lower level of discordance. Mothers with higher socio-economic status, those in higher wealth quintile or more educated, were more likely to report discordance than those with lower socio-economic status. Furthermore, mothers who were never in union were more likely to report discordant PNC than married/living together mothers or those of other marital status. Mothers of children who have died were more likely to report discordance (27% vs 25%).

Table 2 shows the stratification of the analysis by place of birth, distinguishing facility births from non-facility births. The results are similar to those of all births presented in **Table 1** except for woman's education level for which mothers with no education reported higher discordance compared to educated women.

Table 3 presents odds ratios from multivariate logistic regression including all characteristics discussed above for all births and stratified by place of delivery. In the model with all births, delivery in a health facility and receipts of the four ANC interventions are significantly positively associated with PNC discordance (OR = 2.05 and 1.08 respectively). However, delivery with Caesarian section is no longer significant. As shown previously, DHS6 is more likely to show PNC discordance (OR = 1.89) that DHS7. The mother's receipt of PNC is significantly associated with high discordance (OR = 52.3), while the opposite is observed for the newborn (OR = 0.02). Mothers are also likely to report discordant PNC for older newborn, those born 12-23 months before the survey. According to socio-demographic characteristics, mothers with high wealth or education are significantly more like to report discordant PNC. These results are generally maintained when the analysis is stratified by place of residence. For non-facility births, mothers whose children have died and those in other marital status category (divorce or widow) were more likely to report discordant PNC.

DISCUSSION

The journey for a safe and healthy childbirth does not end with the delivery of a healthy newborn but continues during the postnatal period during which mother and newborn are still vulnerable to complications and infections that can lead to morbidity and death. The vulnerability of the postnatal period led the WHO to recommend sequences of health checks post-delivery for

Table 2. *Percentage of mother/newborn by type of discordance with postnatal care (PNC) by socio-demographic and service provision characteristics according to the place of delivery*

CHARACTERISTICS	HEALTH FACILITY DELIVERY				NON-HEALTH FACILITY DELIVERY			
	Discordance, Mom-Yes Baby-No		Discordance, Mom-No Baby-Yes		Discordance, Mom-Yes Baby-No		Discordance, Mom-No Baby-Yes	
	%	95% CI	%	95% CI	%	95% CI	%	95% CI
Age at last birth, category:								
<20	30.6	(29.6, 31.6)	6.1	(5.6, 6.6)	12.5	(11.5, 13.5)	3.9	(3.4, 4.5)
20-34	29.7	(29.2, 30.2)	4.8	(4.6, 5.0)	13.1	(12.5, 13.7)	3.8	(3.6, 4.1)
35+	32.2	(31.0, 33.3)	4.6	(4.1, 5.1)	12.0	(11.1, 13.0)	3.7	(3.2, 4.3)
Months since last birth, category (age of child):								
<6	30.8	(30.0, 31.6)	4.6	(4.3, 4.9)	12.8	(12.0, 13.7)	3.8	(3.3, 4.2)
6-11	30.7	(30.0, 31.5)	5.1	(4.7, 5.5)	12.9	(12.1, 13.7)	3.7	(3.3, 4.1)
12-23	29.5	(28.9, 30.1)	5.1	(4.8, 5.3)	12.8	(12.1, 13.4)	3.9	(3.6, 4.3)
Parity, category								
1	30.2	(29.6, 30.9)	5.1	(4.8, 5.5)	12.9	(12.1, 13.8)	4.4	(3.9, 5.0)
2-3	28.8	(28.2, 29.5)	4.9	(4.6, 5.2)	13.8	(13.1, 14.6)	3.9	(3.5, 4.3)
4+	32.1	(31.3, 32.8)	4.8	(4.5, 5.1)	12.0	(11.3, 12.7)	3.5	(3.2, 3.8)
Months of preceding birth interval, category:								
<24	28	(26.9, 29.1)	4.5	(4.0, 5.0)	11.2	(10.4, 12.2)	4.1	(3.6, 4.8)
24-35	31.9	(31.1, 32.8)	4.4	(4.1, 4.8)	12.5	(11.7, 13.3)	3.7	(3.3, 4.1)
36+	30.5	(29.8, 31.1)	5.2	(4.9, 5.5)	13.3	(12.6, 14.0)	3.6	(3.2, 3.9)
First birth	29.5	(28.8, 30.2)	5.2	(4.8, 5.5)	13.6	(12.7, 14.7)	4.3	(3.8, 5.0)
Wealth quintile combined:								
poorest	28.2	(27.3, 29.1)	5.3	(4.9, 5.8)	11.2	(10.5, 12.0)	3.3	(3.0, 3.7)
poorer	28.9	(28.0, 29.8)	5	(4.6, 5.4)	12.0	(11.3, 12.8)	3.8	(3.4, 4.3)
middle	31.3	(30.4, 32.2)	4.8	(4.5, 5.2)	14.1	(13.1,15.1)	4.2	(3.7, 4.7)
richer	31.7	(30.7, 32.6)	5	(4.6, 5.4)	15.3	(14.1, 16.7)	4	(3.5, 4.7)
richest	30.2	(29.2, 31.3)	4.7	(4.3, 5.1)	17.6	(15.3, 20.1)	5.7	(4.6, 7.1)
Highest educational level:								
no education	37.1	(36.1, 38.1)	3.3	(3.1, 3.6)	11.8	(11.1, 12.5)	3	(2.7, 3.3)
primary	28.6	(27.9, 29.4)	6.1	(5.8, 6.5)	12.4	(11.7, 13.1)	4.3	(3.9, 4.8)
secondary +	28.6	(28.0, 29.2)	4.9	(4.6, 5.2)	16.3	(15.2, 17.4)	5.1	(4.6, 5.8)
Current marital status:								
Never in union	33.3	(31.8, 34.9)	5.6	(4.9, 6.4)	19.7	(17.4, 22.1)	4.9	(3.8, 6.1)
Married/living with partner	30.1	(29.6, 30.6)	4.8	(4.6, 5.0)	12.5	(12.0, 13.0)	3.7	(3.5, 4.0)
Other	26	(24.5, 27.7)	6.3	(5.4, 7.3)	12.9	(10.9, 15.4)	5.2	(4.1, 6.6)
Last birth a caesarean section:								
No	29.0	(28.5, 29.5)	5.3	(5.1, 5.5)	NA		NA	
Yes	36.1	(35.0, 37.1)	3.2	(2.8, 3.7)	NA		NA	
ANC: BP taken + Blood sample + Iron + Urine sample:								
No	26.2	(25.6, 26.8)	5.5	(5.2, 5.8)	9.9	(9.4, 10.4)	3.5	(3.2, 3.7)
Yes	32.7	(32.1, 33.3)	4.6	(4.4, 4.9)	19.4	(18.4, 20.5)	4.6	(4.2, 5.1)
Child is alive:								
No	34.3	(32.3, 36.4)	5.3	(4.1, 6.8)	14.7	(12.7, 16.8)	4.6	(3.6, 5.8)
Yes	30.0	(29.6, 30.5)	4.9	(4.8, 5.1)	12.7	(12.2, 13.3)	3.8	(3.6, 4.0)

CI – confidence interval, ANC – antenatal care, BP – blood pressure

Table 3. *Odds ratio of postnatal care (PNC) discordance between mother and newborn from multivariate logistic regression of all births in the two years preceding the survey, and by place of birth*

Characteristics	All births, N = 280 651		Facility births, N = 198 012		Non-facility births, N = 82 639	
	Odds ratio	95% CI	Odds ratio	95% CI	Odds ratio	95% CI
Age at birth (years):						
<20	1.00		1.00		1.00	
20-35	0.98	(0.94, 1.02)	0.99	(0.94, 1.03)	0.97	(0.88, 1.06)
36+	0.95	(0.90, 1.01)	0.96	(0.90, 1.04)	0.94	(0.83, 1.06)
Parity:						
1 child	1.00		1.00		1.00	
2-3 children	1.01	(0.95, 1.06)	0.99	(0.93, 1.06)	0.98	(0.84, 1.14)
4+ children	1.00	(0.94, 1.06)	0.98	(0.91, 1.05)	0.95	(0.82, 1.11)
Previous birth interval:						
No previous births	1.00		1.00		1.00	
<24 months	0.99	(0.94, 1.04)	0.97	(0.92, 1.03)	1.09	(0.95, 1.26)
24-35 months	0.99	(0.95, 1.04)	0.99	(0.94, 1.04)	1.09	(0.95, 1.25)
36+ months	0.99	(0.95, 1.04)	0.99	(0.95, 1.05)	1.05	(0.91, 1.20)
Wealth quintile:						
Poorest	1.00		1.00		1.00	
2nd poorest	1.04*	(1.01, 1.08)	1.03	(0.99, 1.08)	1.00	(0.94, 1.07)
3rd poorest	1.10*	(1.06, 1.14)	1.06*	(1.01, 1.11)	1.08*	(1.00, 1.16)
4th poorest	1.10*	(1.06, 1.15)	1.07*	(1.02, 1.12)	1.09	(1.00, 1.19)
Least poor	1.06*	(1.01, 1.11)	1.03	(0.98, 1.08)	1.12	(0.99, 1.27)
Woman's education:						
No education	1.00		1.00		1.00	
Primary school	1.13*	(1.09, 1.17)	1.08*	(1.04, 1.13)	1.14*	(1.06, 1.22)
Secondary school+	1.13*	(1.09, 1.17)	1.09*	(1.04, 1.14)	1.16*	(1.08, 1.26)
Woman's marital status:						
Married/living together	1.00		1.00		1.00	
Never in union	1.05	(0.98, 1.12)	1.04	(0.96, 1.12)	1.08	(0.93, 1.25)
Other (divorce, widow)	1.01	(0.95, 1.08)	0.95	(0.88, 1.02)	1.21*	(1.05, 1.39)
Delivered in a facility delivery	2.05*	(1.98, 2.12)	NA		NA	
Survey type, DH6 (ref)	1.89*	(1.65, 2.17)	2.22*	(1.90, 2.59)	1.24	(0.85, 1.81)
Birth was c-section	0.99	(0.95, 1.03)	1.04	(1.00, 1.08)	NA	
Child is currently alive	0.95	(0.89, 1.01)	0.98	(0.90, 1.06)	0.88*	(0.78, 0.99)
Time interval between survey and the delivery (months):						
<6	1.00		1.00		1.00	
6-11	1.03	(1.00, 1.06)	1.03	(0.99, 1.07)	0.99	(0.92, 1.07)
12-23	1.04*	(1.01, 1.07)	1.04*	(1.01, 1.08)	1.01	(0.95, 1.08)
Received 4 ANC components during pregnancy	1.08*	(1.05, 1.11)	1.06*	(1.03, 1.09)	1.15*	(1.08, 1.22)
Mother received postnatal care	52.26*	(50.64, 53.93)	46.93*	(45.26, 48.65)	50.16*	(47.13, 53.39)
Baby received postnatal care	0.02*	(0.02, 0.02)	0.01*	(0.01, 0.02)	0.22*	(0.20, 0.23)

CI – confidence interval, PNC – postnatal care, ANC – antenatal care

*$P < 0.05$. The logistic regressions controlled for specific country.

both the mother and the newborn, regardless of the place of birth, the first being within 24 hours. These health checks are different from care delivered to mothers and newborn during the intrapartum care, for which a separate set of recommendations exist [5].

While the recommendations for PNC appear straightforward, measuring and monitoring the coverage of such contacts continue to be a challenge in low and middle-income countries. These challenges lie in both the design and formulation of PNC questions asked in household surveys and women's recall of these contacts and their timing as distinct from intrapartum care received during delivery in health facilities. Our analysis of 48 DHS implemented since 2011 and covering DHS phases 6 and 7 showed substantial measurement issues that are reflected in the reported coverage of PNC estimates for mothers and newborns. The development of PNC modules in DHS evolved over time both in terms of content of questionnaires and in the target population. We noticed substantial differences in the measurement of PNC for mother and newborn between phases 6 and 7. The content of the questionnaires for PNC newborn differed between DHS 6 and 7, with the later more clarified to improve the understanding of the questions. Such improvements have affected the coverage level of PNC newborn and reduced substantially the level of discordance between mother and newborn in the receipt of PNC. The large gap in the PNC coverage between mother and newborn (42 percentage points on average) and the high level of discordance between mother and newborn in the receipt of PNC (37%) observed in DHS 6 surveys almost disappeared in DHS 7 surveys. In DHS 6 surveys analyzed, PNC mother was estimated at 62% while that of the newborn was 23%. Subsequently, there were 37% discordant PNC between mother and newborn in phase 6, largely in favor of the mother (34%), while only 16% discordant cases were observed in DHS 7 surveys, equally distributed between mother and newborn. Thus, the observed substantial level of PNC discordance between mother and newborn appears driven more by measurement issues than by actual country programs not reaching newborns.

A sensitivity analysis of the reported timing of PNC for mother and newborn in regard to the global PNC indicators based on the first two days after delivery showed that over half of the PNC cases among mothers and newborns were reported to have occurred within the first hour of delivery. This is observed in both phases of the DHS and confirms the continued challenges in distinguishing intrapartum care which often continues up to an hour or more from PNC, and the accurate assessment of the two days following delivery. The reported levels of PNC coverage are therefore substantially overestimated. When PNC that was reported to have occurred within the one hour is considered as no PNC, the coverage levels dropped by half or more regardless of the DHS phase. For DHS 6 surveys analyzed, PNC mother dropped from

62% to 31% and PNC newborn dropped from 31% to 13%. Among DHS 7 surveys, it dropped respectively from 56% to 26% and from 57% to 22%. The size of drop reduced when the reported PNC cases within the first hour were excluded from the data set.

A further assessment of the level and correlates of discordance between PNC mother and newborn showed that women delivering in health facilities were more likely to report discordant PNC between mother and newborn. A total 35% of discordant cases were observed among facility deliveries compared to 16% for non-facility deliveries. This result is primarily because PNC level for non-facility deliveries is low in general. However, the level of discordance among health facility deliveries is concerning and is mostly observed in DHS phase 6 surveys (44% vs 16%) compared to DHS 7 surveys (8% vs 7%). This appears to be due to measurement artifact stemming from questionnaire design and implementation than to programs not reaching mothers and babies.

Our analysis showed that the past and current measurement of PNC for mother and newborn indicators in DHS include substantial measurement errors that challenge the validity of the reported coverage levels across countries, despite some improvements in questionnaires in the latest DHS phases. We have not included data from MICS in the analysis, but past reviews suggested that although coverage gap between mother and newborn is almost inexistent, the very high coverage generally reported may be affected by substantial overestimation due misclassification of intrapartum and immediate essential newborn care as PNC. MICS has adopted a detailed and more stable protocol for PNC measurement since around 2005 The DHS PNC module now follows a similar protocol as MICS but there are still some differences that may affected the comparability of the reported coverage levels.

Measurement errors in PNC contact also come from the recall interviews with mothers. Several studies have shown recall issues from mothers on maternal and newborn health care questions [9-11]. A qualitative study among women in Ghana revealed that mothers can only recall checks that were easily observed and for which the health provider explained the services being provided to the mothers. However, in most cases, mothers are not given any explanation about the care, and sometimes the newborn may be taken away into another room for care. [12] In Malawi and Bangladesh, women could not understand the health check questions, prompting DHS to revise the PNC questions to include example of health check. However, there remains a substantial confusion between intrapartum care and PNC visits [13]. Observation-based validation studies in Kenya and Swaziland have also demonstrated issues with women's recall of care received during postnatal period [14,15].

The current global PNC trends databases based on DHS and MICS and other national surveys cannot be used to accurately capture trends in PNC coverage that are reflective of maternal and newborn health program and service delivery in countries. Further assessm ent and validation of measurement procedures are urgently warranted. Such initiatives must also consider the current gap in measuring the joint PNC of mother and newborn to support the desire to promote focus on both mother and newborn together.

Funding: *Bill & Melinda Gates Foundation. The funder had no role in the writing of this manuscript.*

Authorship contributions: *AA conceived the paper, developed the analysis plan, supervised the analysis, and wrote the initial draft. EH carried out the analysis and contributed to the write up of the initial draft. LV, YS, AM reviewed, edited and commented on the initial drafts. All authors reviewed all drafts and approved the final manuscript.*

Competing interests: *The authors completed the ICMJE Unified Competing Interest form (available upon request from the corresponding author), and declare no conflicts of interest.*

Additional material
Online Supplementary Document

References
1 Baqui AH, Ahmed S, El Arifeen S, Darmstadt GL, Rosecrans AM, Mannan I, et al. Effect of timing of first postnatal care home visit on neonatal mortality in Bangladesh: a observational cohort study. BMJ. 2009;339:b2826. Medline:19684100 doi:10.1136/bmj.b2826

2 Baqui AH, Arifeen SE, Williams EK, Ahmed S, Mannan I, Rahman SM, et al. Effectiveness of home-based management of newborn infections by community health workers in rural Bangladesh. Pediatr Infect Dis J. 2009;28:304-10. Medline:19289979 doi:10.1097/INF.0b013e31819069e8

3 Bhutta ZA, Das JK, Bahl R, Lawn JE, Salam RA, Paul VK, et al. Can available interventions end preventable deaths in mothers, newborn babies, and stillbirths, and at what cost? Lancet. 2014;384:347-70. Medline:24853604 doi:10.1016/S0140-6736(14)60792-3

4 World Health Organization. WHO recommendations on postnatal care of mother and newborn (2013). Geneva: World Health Organization; 2014.

5 World Health Organization. WHO recommendation. Intrapartum care for a positive childbirth experience. Geneva: World Health Organization; 2018.

6 Moran AC, Kerber K, Sitrin D, Guenther T, Morrissey CS, Newby H, et al. Measuring coverage in MNCH: indicators for global tracking of newborn care. PLoS Med. 2013;10:e1001415. Medline:23667335 doi:10.1371/journal.pmed.1001415

7 Amouzou A, Mehra V, Carvajal-Aguirre L, Khan SM, Sitrin D, Vaz LM. Measuring postnatal care contacts for mothers and newborns: An analysis of data from the MICS and DHS surveys. J Glob Health. 2017;7:020502. Medline:29423179 doi:10.7189/jogh.07.020502

8 Countdown to 2030 Collaboration. Countdown to 2030: tracking progress towards universal coverage for reproductive, maternal, newborn, and child health. Lancet. 2018;391:1538-48. Medline:29395268 doi:10.1016/S0140-6736(18)30104-1

9 Blanc AK, Warren C, McCarthy KJ, Kimani J, Ndwiga C. RamaRao S. Assessing the validity of indicators of the quality of maternal and newborn health care in Kenya. J Glob Health. 2016;6:010405. Medline:27231541 doi:10.7189/jogh.06.010405

10 Blanc AK, Diaz C, McCarthy KJ, Berdichevsky K. Measuring progress in maternal and newborn health care in Mexico: validating indicators of health system contact and quality of care. BMC Pregnancy Childbirth. 2016;16:255. Medline:27577266 doi:10.1186/s12884-016-1047-0

11 Stanton CK, Rawlins B, Drake M, Dos Anjos M, Cantor D, Chongo L, et al. Measuring coverage in MNCH: testing the validity of women's self-report of key maternal and newborn health interventions during the peripartum period in Mozambique. PLoS One. 2013;8:e60694. Medline:23667427 doi:10.1371/journal.pone.0060694

12 Hill Z, Okyere E, Wickenden M, Tawiah-Agyemang C. What can we learn about post-natal care in Ghana if we ask the right questions? A qualitative study. Glob Health Action. 2015;8:28515. Medline:26350434 doi:10.3402/gha.v8.28515

13 Yoder PS, Rosato M, Mahmud R, Fort A, Rahman F, Armstrong A, et al. Women's revall of delivery and neonatal care in Bangladesh and Malawi. Calverton, Maryland, USA: ICF Macro, 2010.

14 McCarthy KJ, Blanc AK, Warren CE, Mdawida B. Women's recall of maternal and newborn interventions received in the postnatal period: a validity study in Kenya and Swaziland. J Glob Health. 2018;8:010605. Medline:29904605 doi:10.7189/jogh.08.010605

15 McCarthy KJ, Blanc AK, Warren CE, Kimani J, Mdawida B, Ndwidga C. Can surveys of women accurately track indicators of maternal and newborn care? A validity and reliability study in Kenya. J Glob Health. 2016;6:020502. Medline:27606061 doi:10.7189/jogh.06.020502

Variance estimation for effective coverage measures: A simulation study

Sara M Sauer[1], Thomas Pullum[2], Wenjuan Wang[2,3*], Lindsay Mallick[4], Hannah H Leslie[5]

[1] Department of Biostatistics, Harvard T.H. Chan School of Public Health, Boston, Massachusetts, USA

[2] The Demographic and Health Surveys (DHS) Program, Division of International Health and Development, ICF, Rockville, Maryland, USA

[3] Division of AIDS, Behavioral, and Population Sciences; Center for Scientific Review, National Institutes of Health; Bethesda, Maryland, USA

[4] The DHS Program, Avenir Health; Glastonbury, Connecticut, USA

[5] Department of Global Health and Population, Harvard T.H. Chan School of Public Health, Boston, Massachusetts, USA

* This work was prepared while Wenjuan Wang was employed at ICF. The opinions expressed in this article are the author's own and do not reflect the view of the National Institutes of Health, the Department of Health and Human Services, or the United States government.

Background Effective coverage research is increasing rapidly in global health and development, as researchers use a range of measures and combine data sources to adjust coverage for the quality of services received. However, most estimates of effective coverage that combine data sources are reported only as point estimates, which may be due to the challenge of calculating the variance for a composite measure. In this paper, we evaluate three methods to quantify the uncertainty in the estimation of effective coverage.

Methods We conducted a simulation study to evaluate the performance of the exact, delta, and parametric bootstrap methods for constructing confidence intervals around point estimates that are calculated from combined data on coverage and quality. We assessed performance by computing the number of nominally 95% confidence intervals that contain the truth for a range of coverage and quality values and data source sample sizes. To illustrate these approaches, we applied the delta and exact methods to estimates of adjusted coverage of antenatal care (ANC) in Senegal. We used household survey data for coverage and health facility assessments for readiness to provide services.

Results With small sample sizes, when the true effective coverage value was close to the boundaries 0 or 1, the exact and parametric bootstrap methods resulted in substantial over or undercoverage and, for the exact method, a high proportion of invalid confidence intervals, while the delta method yielded modest overcoverage. The proportion of confidence intervals containing the truth in all three methods approached the intended 95% with larger sample sizes and as the true effective coverage value moved away from the 0 or 1 boundary. Confidence intervals for adjusted ANC in Senegal were largely overlapping across the delta and exact methods, although at the sub-national level, the exact method produced invalid confidence intervals for estimates near 0 or 1. We provide the code to implement these methods.

Conclusions The uncertainty around an effective coverage estimate can be characterized; this should become standard practice if effective coverage estimates are to become part of national and global health monitoring. The delta method approach outperformed the other methods in this study; we recommend its use for appropriate inference from effective coverage estimates that combine data sources, particularly when either sample size is small. When used for estimates created from facility type or regional strata, these methods require assumptions of independence that must be considered in each example.

Progress towards global development goals, including Sustainable Development Goal (SDG) 3: good health and well-being, is dependent on the operation of complex systems in both high and low-resource settings [1]. Achieving the ambitious health targets in Goal 3 demands that health systems, in order to successfully manage population health, must prevent disease, treat acute and chronic illness, and respond to emergencies and disasters [2].

While global monitoring early in the 2000s focused on health system coverage and the proportion of those in need who receive a service, there is increasing recognition that monitoring in the SDG era must evaluate the effectiveness of service in order to capture the true value of health systems [3,4]. This is reflected in the growing research on effective coverage of health interventions [5]. Effective coverage can be defined as the fraction of potential health gain successfully delivered [3], or more operationally, as the "people who need health services obtain[ing] them in a timely manner and at a level of quality necessary to obtain the desired effect and potential health gains" [6].

Effective coverage research is increasing rapidly in global health, as researchers use a range of measures to adjust coverage for the quality and effects of care received [5]. The calculation of measures of effective coverage frequently requires combining data from different sources, such as administrative records that provide service coverage and clinic data for the content or quality of services [7]. A recent review and framework for effective coverage recommended reserving the term "effective coverage" for outcome-adjusted coverage and specifying input-adjusted or process-adjusted coverage based on the type of measure used for service delivery [5]. Here we use "effective coverage" generally for any adjusted coverage estimate, given its use in existing literature, and refer to specific estimates as suggested in this framework.

As an example, multiple studies have attempted to quantify quality-adjusted coverage of antenatal care (ANC). All pregnant women are encouraged to attend formal health care during pregnancy for assessment, preventive measures, and counseling. The focused ANC model recommended by the World Health Organization (WHO) in 2002 included four visits for basic care, with the first visit taking place ideally within the first 12 weeks of gestation [8]. The Millennium Development Goal to improve maternal health included attendance at four ANC visits as a key target for service coverage [9]. In 2016, the WHO released guidelines that increased the recommended contacts to eight [10], although this has not yet been widely adopted as a measure of coverage. Studies on quality-adjusted coverage have used both one visit and four visits to quantify ANC coverage, which is based typically on maternal self-report in household surveys [11-19]. Facility measures have similarly followed WHO guidance on the expectations for ANC and have generally focused on inputs to care, with studies that define structural quality measures for health facilities such as functional diagnostics and medications [11,15,16]. Across all studies, despite the variation in measurement, crude coverage of ANC substantially exceeded the adjusted coverage. Failing to consider either facility readiness or quality of care can dramatically overstate health system performance.

Multinational and academic groups have called for a transition from coverage measures to effective coverage measures in order to appropriately benchmark and monitor national progress towards the SDGs [2,4,20]. Effective coverage metrics require accurate estimation of uncertainty around each estimate. While it is routine to report variance for effective coverage estimates that use one data source [19,21,22], most research that integrates multiple data sources to estimate effective coverage provides only point estimates. A 2018 literature review [5] found that of six papers that combined population and health facility data sources, four did not report an estimate of the variance of the point estimate [11,12,15,16]; one used the exact method for the product of two variables [17], and the sixth used a Taylor series expansion [19]. Recently published work on the effective coverage of childbirth defined and employed the delta method for variance calculation [23,24].

This paper aims to provide a formal definition of effective coverage; describe the exact, delta, and bootstrap methods of constructing confidence intervals around effective coverage estimates; test the methods' performance with a simulation study; demonstrate their application to the estimation of effective coverage of ANC in Senegal; and provide guidance for applied research.

METHODS

Effective coverage can be defined at three levels: *first*, for a specific combination of facility type f and region r; *second*, for region r, combining all facility types; *third*, at the national level, combining all regions. When combining two data sources without an exact link between individuals and health facilities, incorporating health facility type improves the accuracy of the overall estimates [25]. Here we present the analytical approaches for all three levels. We conducted the simulations at a single level to demonstrate method performance in the most simple setting.

Calculating effective coverage

Estimates of effective coverage are specific to a particular type of intervention. For example, an intervention could be ANC for recently pregnant women age 15-49, and the relevant readiness measure could be a binary or continuous measure of facility preparedness to offer high-quality ANC. For illustration, we define a binary random variable X_{rf} that represents crude coverage and a binary random variable Y_{rf} that represents facility readiness, both of which are specific to sub-national region r and facility type f. (The full derivation of effective coverage is shown in Appendix S1 of the **Online Supplementary Document**). The distributions of these random variables are indexed by a mean parameter $P(X_{rf}=1)=P_{xrf}$ and $P(Y_{rf}=1)=P_{yrf}$, respectively. Since P_{xrf} and P_{yrf} are usually unknown in practice, these probabilities are estimated with sample means. Let p_{xrf} be the estimated measure of coverage, such as the sample proportion of women who seek ANC in facilities of type f in region r. Let p_{yrf} be the estimated measure of readiness, such as the sample proportion of facilities of type f in region r that satisfy minimal criteria for ANC. The estimated effective coverage p_{rf} for this combination of r and f is a product:

$$p_{rf}=p_{xrf}\times p_{yrf} \tag{1}$$

At the regional level, the effective coverage p_r is obtained by adding the contributions from all facilities:

$$p_r=\Sigma_f p_{rf} \tag{2}$$

This can also be viewed as a weighted sum of readiness p_{yrf} where the weights are the proportion of women attending that facility type $(p_{xrf}, \Sigma_f \times p_{rf}=1)$. The national effective coverage p is a weighted average of the regional values. The weights w_r $(\Sigma_r \times w_r=1)$ are proportional to the relevant denominator for each region, such as the number of women or the number of pregnancies:

$$P=\Sigma_r w_r p_r \tag{3}$$

Calculating a confidence interval for effective coverage

We describe three methods for constructing a 95% confidence interval around an effective coverage estimate: two analytical approaches, the *exact* and the *delta* methods, and a computer-based approach, the *bootstrap* method, which involves repeated sampling with parameters estimated from the observed data. The derivation for confidence interval construction using the *delta* method was presented previously in Wang et al. [23,26].

Method 1: The exact method

The exact method of calculating the sampling variance of effective coverage estimates is based on a formula for the exact variance of the product of two independent random variables derived by Goodman in 1960 [27]. By definition, the variance of the product of two random variables Z and M is $Var(ZM) = E[(ZM)^2] - (E[ZM])^2$. If the two variables are independent, then $E[Z^2M^2] = E[Z^2] E[M^2]$ and $E[ZM] = E[Z] E[M]$, from which it follows that $Var(ZM) = E[Z^2] E[M^2] - (E[Z] E[M])^2$. Since $E[Z^2] = Var(Z) + E[Z]^2$, and $E[M^2] = Var(M) + E[M]^2$, $Var(ZM)$ can be re-expressed as

$$Var(ZM) = (Var(Z) + E[Z]^2) \times (Var(M) + E[M]^2) - (E[Z] E[M])^2 \tag{4}.$$

This formula can be used to calculate the variance of $p_{rf} = p_{xrf} \times p_{yrf}$ denoted by $se^2(p_{rf})$:

$$se^2(p_{rf}) = [Var(p_{xrf}) + E[p_{xrf}]^2] [Var(p_{yrf}) + E[p_{yrf}]^2] - E[p_{rf}]^2 \tag{5}$$

Assuming a normal approximation to the distributions of p_{xrf} and p_{xrf} yields $Var(p_{xrf}) = (P_{xrf}(1-P_{xrf}))/n_{xrf}$ and $Var(p_{yrf}) = (P_{yrf}(1-P_{yrf}))/n_{yrf}$ where n_{xrf} and n_{yrf} are the sample sizes if the samples were collected via simple random sampling, or the effective sample sizes, if the samples were collected through a complex survey design. These quantities can be estimated using p_{xrf} and p_{yrf} in place of P_{xrf} and P_{yrf} respectively. The *estimated* variance of $p_{rf} = p_{xrf} p_{yrf}$ denoted by $s^2(p_{rf})$, is then given by:

$$s^2(p_{rf}) = [(p_{xrf}(1-p_{xrf}))/n_{xrf} + p^2_{xrf}][(p_{yrf}(1-p_{yrf}))/n_{yrf} + p^2_{yrf}] - p^2_{rf} \tag{6}$$

The approach under the exact method is to calculate the estimated standard error $s_{rf} = s(p_{rf})$ using (6), and then use a normal approximation to the distribution of p_{rf} to calculate

$$L_{prf} = p_{rf} - 1.96 s_{rf} \text{ and } U_{prf} = p_{rf} + 1.96 s_{rf} \tag{7}.$$

as the lower and upper ends, respectively, of the 95% confidence interval for effective coverage.

To summarize, this method is exact in equations (4) and (5); equation (6) provides an estimate of the variance based on observed sample proportions; and (7) gives a symmetric Wald-type 95% confidence interval. When p_{rf} is close to either 0 or 1, it is possible for this confidence interval to cross the 0,1 boundary and yield an invalid confidence interval.

Expression (6) can be modified to take into account the facility and regional levels as follows:

$$s^2_{rf} = [(p_{xrf}(1-p_{xrf}))/n_{xrf} + p^2_{xrf}] \, [(p_{yrf}(1-p_{yrf}))/n_{yrf} + p^2_{yrf}] - p^2_{rf}$$

$$s^2_{r} = \Sigma_f [(p_{xrf}(1-p_{xrf}))/n_{xrf} + p^2_{xrf}] \, [(p_{yrf}(1-p_{yrf}))/n_{yrf} + p^2_{yrf}] - p^2_{rf}$$

$$s^2 = \Sigma_f w^2_r \, \Sigma_f [(p_{xrf}(1-p_{xrf}))/n_{xrf} + p^2_{xrf}] \, [(p_{yrf} \, (1-p_{yrf}))/n_{yrf} + p^2_{yrf}] - p^2_{rf}$$

Note that we assume independence (covariance = 0) between the effective coverage estimates for different facility/regional levels in the expressions above (as well as in the following methods). This is an assumption that should be evaluated in each application of these methods.

Method 2: The delta method

An alternative approach to constructing a 95% confidence interval for a proportion is to transform the proportion to a logit scale, calculate the confidence interval on that scale, and then take antilogits of the confidence interval endpoints to return to the original scale. Specifically, consider the proportion P, which is estimated by p. Define

$$F = logit(p) = b \tag{8}.$$

In this representation, b is the intercept or constant term from a logit regression with no covariates. Let s_b be the standard error of b. Under the assumption that b, rather than p, has a normal sampling distribution, a 95% confidence interval for the population value of b with lower and upper limits L_F and U_F, respectively, is calculated as

$$L_F = F - 1.96s_b \text{ and } U_F = F + 1.96s_b \tag{9}.$$

We calculate the inverse transformation of the logit, or the antilogit, to obtain the lower and upper limits of the 95% confidence interval for P:

$$L = exp(L_F)/[1 + exp(L_F)] \text{ and } U = exp(U_F)/[1 + exp(U_F)] \tag{10}.$$

If n_0 and n_1 are the number of cases with $X = 0$ and $X = 1$, respectively, then $b = log(n_1/n_0)$ and $s_b = sqrt[(1/n_0) + (1/n_1)]$. Standard statistical software will produce b, s_b, L_F, and U_F, and can adjust for sample weights, clustering, and stratification, if applicable.

When p represents the effective coverage estimate, we cannot use an exact formula to calculate s_b, the standard error of $logit(p)$, because $logit(p)$ cannot be factored into a product of two variables. We can, however, calculate the b's and s's from the readiness and coverage data separately, and use these to approximate s_b. Suppose that b_x and b_y are the intercepts from logit regressions of X and Y separately, with sampling s^2_{bx} and s^2_{by}, respectively, all of which are produced with standard statistical packages. If $F = F(b_x, b_y)$ is a joint function of b_x and b_y, then an approximation to the sampling variance of F is given by

$$s^2 = \left(\frac{\partial F}{\partial b_x}\right)^2 s_{bx}^2 + \left(\frac{\partial F}{\partial b_y}\right)^2 s_{by}^2 = \sum_{k=x}^{y}\left(\frac{\partial F}{\partial b_k}\right)^2 s_{bk}^2 \tag{11}.$$

This well-known approximation is sometimes described as the delta method [28].

Now we apply the delta method to the logit of effective coverage. The logit transformation is applied to three levels of effective coverage: *first*, for facility type f in region r; *second*, for region r; and *third*, at the national level, for which no subscripts are needed. The transformations are

$$F_{rf} = logit(p_{rf}) \tag{12}.$$

$$F_r = logit(p_r) \tag{13}.$$

$$F = logit(p) \tag{14}.$$

At these three levels, (11) takes the following forms:

$$s_{brf}^2 = \sum_{k=y}^{x}\left(\frac{\partial F_{rf}}{\partial b_{krf}}\right)^2 s_{bkrf}^2 \tag{15}.$$

$$s_{br}^2 = \sum_{f}\sum_{k=y}^{x}\left(\frac{\partial F_r}{\partial b_{bkrf}}\right)^2 s_{bkrf}^2 \tag{16}.$$

$$s_b^2 = \sum_{r}\sum_{f}\sum_{k=y}^{x}\left(\frac{\partial F}{\partial b_{krf}}\right)^2 s_{bkrf}^2 \tag{17}.$$

The components for the chained partial derivatives are provided in Appendix S2 of the **Online Supplementary Document**. When the components are multiplied together as described, the partial derivatives required for equations (15), (16), and (17) are given by (18), (19), and (20), respectively:

$$\frac{\partial F_{rf}}{\partial b_{krf}} = \left(1 - p_{krf}\right) / \left(1 - p_{rf}\right) \tag{18}.$$

$$\frac{\partial F_r}{\partial b_{krf}} = p_{rf}\left(1 - p_{krf}\right) / \left[p_r\left(1 - p_r\right)\right] \tag{19}.$$

$$\frac{\partial F}{\partial b_{krf}} = w_r p_{rf}\left(1 - p_{krf}\right) / \left[p\left(1 - p\right)\right] \tag{20}.$$

To summarize this approach, partial derivatives are calculated from (18) or (19) or (20). The s's are produced by logit regression software. At each level, a confidence interval is constructed for F, and the endpoints of that interval are converted to a confidence interval (L, U) for P by taking antilogits, as in (10).

In some cases, facility readiness may be a continuous score rather than a binary measure. **Figure 1** summarizes the variance calculations for the exact and delta methods in the case of a binary coverage indicator and a binary or

	Delta method: $antilogit(F \pm 1.96 \times s_{b_{rf}})$, where $s_{b_{rf}}^2 =$	Exact method: $p \pm 1.96 s_{rf}$, where $s_{rf}^2 =$
Binary coverage indicator / Binary readiness indicator	$\sum_{k=y}^{x} \left(\frac{\partial F_{rf}}{\partial b_{krf}}\right)^2 s_{b_{krf}}^2$, with $\frac{\partial F_{rf}}{\partial b_{krf}} = (1 - p_{krf})/(1 - p_{rf})$	$[(p_{xrf}(1 - p_{xrf}))/n_{xrf}$ $+ p_{xrf}^2][(p_{yrf}(1 - p_{yrf}))/n_{yrf}$ $+ p_{yrf}^2] - p_{rf}^2$
Binary coverage indicator / Continuous readiness score	$\sum_{k=y}^{x} \left(\frac{\partial F_{rf}}{\partial b_{krf}}\right)^2 s_{b_{krf}}^2$, with $\frac{\partial F_{rf}}{\partial b_{yrf}} = 1/[p_{yrf}(1 - p_{rf})]$ and $\frac{\partial F_{rf}}{\partial b_{xrf}} = (1 - p_{xrf})/(1 - p_{rf})$	$[(p_{xrf}(1 - p_{xrf}))/n_{xrf}$ $+ p_{xrf}^2][[\frac{1}{n_{yrf}}(\frac{\sum_i(Y_{irf} - \overline{Y}_{rf})^2}{(n_{yrf} - 1)})]$ $+ p_{yrf}^2] - p_{rf}^2$

Figure 1. *Delta and exact methods for construction of a 95% confidence interval around the effective coverage estimate for a specific facility type f in a specific region r, prf.*

a continuous readiness measure. Details of the modifications to the formulas in the case of a continuous readiness measure are shown in Appendix S3 of the **Online Supplementary Document**.

Method 3: The bootstrap method

The final approach we consider is a bootstrap method, a computer-based approach that involves repeated sampling from a distribution or the observed data [29]. Bootstrapping methods are used increasingly to generate variance estimates for complex parameters. We first compared a non-parametric bootstrap in which observations are re-sampled from observed data (with replacement) to a parametric bootstrap in which observations are generated with parameters estimated from the original sample. Initial comparisons revealed consistent undercoverage when using a nonparametric bootstrap. We therefore focus on the parametric bootstrap for the full analysis. When coverage and readiness are proportions as presented above, the steps for constructing a 95% confidence interval for the effective coverage estimate for a particular region r and facility type f based on a simple random sample for each data source are as follows:

- Obtain p_{xrf} and p_{yrf} from the observed data,
- Use these estimates to generate B samples from Binomial(n_{xrf}, p_{xrf}), and B samples from Binomial(n_{yrf}, p_{yrf}),
- Divide the sampled values by n_{xrf} and n_{yrf} respectively to get the B-vectors p_{xrf_boot} and p_{yrf_boot},
- Multiply the corresponding elements of p_{xrf_boot} and p_{yrf_boot} to get the B-vector p_{boot},
- Obtain the upper and lower limits of the 95% confidence interval using the 2.5th and 97.5th percentiles of the distribution of p_{boot}.

If readiness is a continuous score, this procedure can be modified to generate data using an appropriate distribution.

Simulation study

We designed a simulation study to test the performance of the confidence interval construction methods in settings with small and modest sample sizes. In many cases in applied research, the sample size for health facilities will be much smaller than the individual sample. We tested settings of both equal and unequal sample sizes.

We assume that the crude coverage of a service in the population is a binary measure with probability P_{xrf} and health system quality is a binary measure with probability P_{yrf}. We test combinations of P_{xrf} and P_{yrf} over the range (0.02, 0.98) and with sample sizes for n_{xrf} the number of individuals sampled, and n_{yrf} the number of facilities sampled, that varied between 50 and 500 (all settings considered are presented in **Table 1**). In each case, the sample of individuals and the sample of facilities are simple random samples. As a further analysis, we consider the case in which the service readiness measure is a continuous score on 0,1.

Table 1. *Simulation settings*

Term	Definition	Simulation settings
P_{xrf}	Proportion of individuals in need accessing service (crude coverage)	(0.02, 0.04, 0.06, 0.08, 0.1, 0.15, 0.2, 0.25, 0.30, 0.35, 0.40, 0.45, 0.50, 0.55, 0.6, 0.65, 0.70, 0.75, 0.80, 0.85, 0.90, 0.92, 0.94, 0.96, 0.98)
P_{yrf}	Proportion of health facilities rated as 'high-quality'	(0.02, 0.04, 0.06, 0.08, 0.1, 0.15, 0.2, 0.25, 0.30, 0.35, 0.40, 0.45, 0.50, 0.55, 0.6, 0.65, 0.70, 0.75, 0.80, 0.85, 0.90, 0.92, 0.94, 0.96, 0.98)
n_{xrf}	Number of individuals sampled	(n_{xrf}, n_{yrf}) = (50, 50), (100, 100), (200, 200), (300, 300), (400, 400),
n_{yrf}	Number of facilities sampled	(500, 500), (100, 50), (200, 50), (300, 50), (400, 50), (500, 50)

For each simulation setting, we generated 10 000 data sets. For each simulated data set, we computed the effective coverage estimate $p_{rf} = p_{xrf} p_{yrf}$ and constructed 95% confidence intervals around p_{rf} using the exact, delta, and bootstrap methods. For the bootstrap method, 10 000 bootstrap samples were taken to construct the confidence interval at each iteration. Across the 10 000 simulated iterations, we calculated the estimated coverage probabilities of the three methods for constructing a 95% confidence interval by computing the proportion of iterations in which the true effective coverage value was contained in the 95% confidence interval. When computing the estimated coverage probabilities for the exact and bootstrap methods, we removed the iterations that resulted in a degenerate confidence interval, which occurs when

$p_{rf}=0$ or 1. When estimating the coverage probabilities for the delta method, we removed the iterations that resulted in an undefined confidence interval, which occurs when when $p_{rf}=0$ or when either p_{xrf} or $p_{yrf}=1$. We recorded the number of undefined confidence intervals for the delta method, which is the maximum number of iterations removed across the three methods, and the number of invalid estimates for the exact method (the instances in which the confidence interval bounds fall below 0 or above 1).

Applied example

We demonstrate the application of these methods using real data on ANC coverage and facility readiness in the Republic of Senegal. The West African nation of Senegal is home to over 13 million individuals who live in 14 administrative regions [30]. Senegal is classified as a low-income country by the World Bank. The public health sector is organized into hospitals at the top, followed by intermediate health centers and peripheral health posts. Health extension huts (*cases de santé*) offer limited services, which are largely for reproductive, maternal, and child health, while the private sector also provides health services. From 2012 to 2017, the National Agency for Statistics and Demography partnered with ICF International to implement a simultaneous and continuous Demographic and Health Survey (DHS) and Service Provision Assessment (SPA). Each assessment was administered annually over the 5-year period. We relied on the 2017 surveys, using the DHS to define coverage and the SPA to define readiness.

The DHS is a population-based household sample, in which women age 15 to 49 answer questions about their reproductive history. We defined ANC coverage based on responses from women with a live birth in the past 2 years, and calculated three measures based on global and national standards of care:

- **Coverage 1**: self-report of any ANC with a formal health care provider

- **Coverage 4**: self-report of 4 or more ANC visits

- **Coverage 8**: self-report of 8 or more ANC visits

The SPA is a health facility assessment that includes an audit of service availability and readiness, as well as provider interviews and observations of care. We use the facility audit to define readiness to provide high-quality ANC, which was limited to health facilities that provide ANC. To best illustrate the variance estimation methods, we defined two binary indicators (one prevalent, one rare) and a bounded score as quality measures:

- **Readiness 1**: Availability of manual or digital blood pressure apparatus (binary)

- **Readiness 2**: Availability of hemoglobin and urine protein diagnostic capacity (binary)

- **Readiness 3**: ANC service readiness, the proportion of essential inputs in place across four domains as defined by the WHO: basic amenities (guidelines, visual aids, and provider training); equipment (manual or digital blood pressure apparatus); diagnostics (urine and anemia testing capacity); and medication (iron and folic acid, tetanus toxoid, and IPTp and ITNs for malaria) [31]. We weighted items evenly within domain and domains equally within the score.

To define adjusted coverage, we calculated service readiness by strata defined by the fourteen regions and five health facility types (government hospital, government health center, government health clinic/post, private hospital/ health center/clinic, health hut). Coverage was estimated for the same strata. In this example, we assigned women who identified multiple sources of care the source with the highest readiness and assumed that all visits took place at that source or a similar source. This will overestimate adjusted coverage for women using multiple sources of care of varying readiness. We calculated adjusted coverage as the product of coverage and readiness within strata and estimated national adjusted coverage as the average of stratum-specific estimates weighted by population size (women reporting live births in the previous 2 years).

We repeated this procedure for the nine combinations of the coverage and quality measures and used the exact and delta methods to quantify variance in each case. The complex sample designs used for both DHS and SPA are accounted for by using the survey setting. For the DHS, the strata are based on sub-national region and urban/rural residence; the cluster is the primary sampling unit, and individual weights are the women's sampling weight that account for non-response and sampling probability. For the SPA, the strata are based on sub-national region, health facility type, and managing authority; the primary sampling unit is the facility, and the individual weights are the facility sampling weight. Although the bootstrap method, particularly the non-parametric bootstrap, can be modified for complex survey data [32], expanding the parametric bootstrap method for a parameter derived from two complex surveys is beyond the scope of this paper and is an area for future research.

Simulations were conducted in R (The R Foundation for Statistical Computing, Vienna, Austria). Applied analyses were conducted with Stata version 15 (StataCorp, College Station, Texas, USA). A program for calculating point estimates and confidence intervals in Stata for national and sub-national analyses like the applied example as well as sub-sample analyses to assess equity is included in the **Online Supplementary Document** and at this link (https://osf.io/9nsaf/?view_only=681d595548014a17a4a666690e708336), as is the simulation code in R.

Ethical approval

The original survey implementers obtained ethical approvals for data collection; the Harvard University Research Protection Program deemed this analysis exempt from human subjects review.

RESULTS

Simulation study

The simulation results for the estimated coverage probabilities are shown in **Figure 2**, **Figure 3**, and **Figure 4** for the exact, delta, and bootstrap methods, respectively. The maximum proportion of simulations with undefined estimates is shown in Appendix S4 in the **Online Supplementary Document**.

When the sample size is small, and when the true proportions P_{xrf} and/or P_{yrf} are close to 0 or 1, the confidence intervals constructed using the exact method result in severe overcoverage for the most extreme values of P_{xrf} and P_{yrf} which then becomes undercoverage as P_{xrf} and P_{yrf} increase. Of the iterations that do not result in degenerate confidence intervals, the nominally 95% confidence interval captures the truth 100% of the time in the extreme case of $P_{xrf} = 0.02$ and $P_{yrf} = 0.02$ with $(n_{xrf}, n_{yrf}) = (50, 50)$, as shown in **Figure 2**, Panel A. Moreover, as shown in Appendix S4 of the **Online Supplementary Document**, all of the non-degenerate confidence intervals constructed in this setting are invalid, with the lower bound falling below 0. For small sample sizes and values of P_{xrf} and P_{yrf} between 0.06 and 0.25, the exact method yielded confidence intervals that contained the truth closer to 90 than 95% of the time. This undercoverage may be due to the use of a normal approximation, which may not be valid with small sample sizes. A similar pattern persists at sample sizes of 100 (**Figure 2**, Panels B and C). When both n_{xrf} and n_{yrf} are 500, the coverage is generally at or close to the nominal level (0.95), except for very extreme values of P_{xrf} or P_{yrf} (**Figure 2**, Panel D).

The confidence intervals constructed with the delta method yield estimated coverage probabilities that are generally close to the nominal level of 95%, although for small sample sizes and extreme values of P_{xrf} or P_{yrf} this method results in overcoverage as high as 98% (**Figure 3**, Panel A). Coverage is uniformly close to the nominal 95% level once sample sizes reach 400 to 500.

The results for the bootstrap method mirror those described for the exact method, with slightly better performance compared to the exact method. In

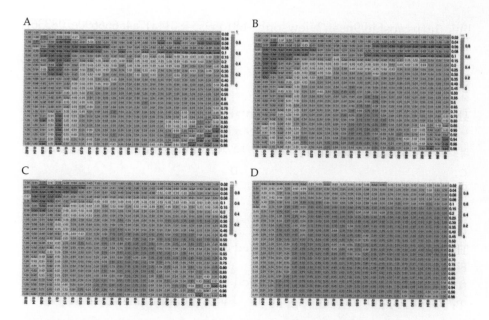

Figure 2. *Estimated 95% coverage probabilities for the confidence intervals constructed using the exact method. P_{xrf} and P_{yrf} vary over the range (0.02, 0.98).* **Panel A.** *(n_{xrf} n_{yrf}) = (50, 50).* **Panel B.** *(n_{xrf} n_{yrf}) = (100, 50).* **Panel C.** *(n_{xrf} n_{yrf}) = (100, 100).* **Panel D.** *(n_{xrf} n_{yrf}) = (500, 500).*

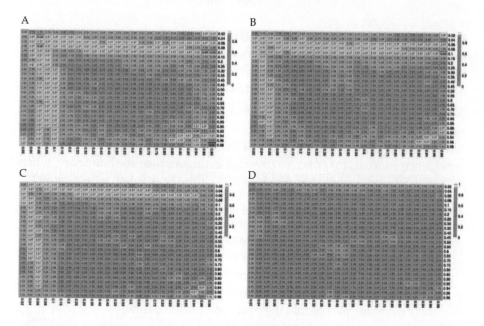

Figure 3. *Estimated 95% coverage probabilities for the confidence intervals constructed using the delta method. P_{xrf} and P_{yrf} vary over the range (0.02, 0.98).* **Panel A.** *(n_{xrf} n_{yrf}) = (50, 50).* **Panel B.** *(n_{xrf} n_{yrf}) = (100, 50).* **Panel C.** *(n_{xrf} n_{yrf}) = (100, 100).* **Panel D.** *(n_{xrf} n_{yrf}) = (500, 500).*

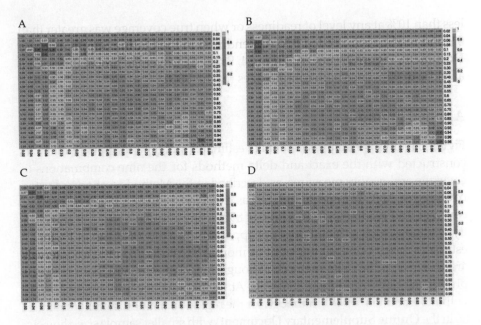

Figure 4. *Estimated 95% coverage probabilities for the confidence intervals constructed using the parametric bootstrap method. P_{xrf} and P_{yrf} vary over the range (0.02, 0.98).* **Panel A.** *(n_{xrf} n_{yrf}) = (50, 50).* **Panel B.** *(n_{xrf} n_{yrf}) = (100, 50).* **Panel C.** *(n_{xrf} n_{yrf}) = (100, 100).* **Panel D.** *(n_{xrf} n_{yrf}) = (500, 500).*

particular, we see overcoverage (99-100%) for small sample sizes and very extreme values of P_{xrf} or P_{yrf} which then becomes undercoverage for values of P_{xrf} and P_{yrf} up to approximately 0.25 (**Figure 4**, Panel A). With samples of at least 500, coverage is no lower than 92% (**Figure 4**, Panel D).

Appendix S4 in the **Online Supplementary Document** includes full results with the number of invalid confidence interval bounds for the exact method, which occurred in as high as 100% of the iterations yielding non-degenrate confidence intervals for effective coverage estimates near the boundary, when $n_{xrf} = n_{yrf} = 50$, and occurred as much as 26% of the time when $n_{xrf} = n_{yrf} = 500$.

When using a continuous score as a readiness estimate instead of a binary indicator, the relative performance of the confidence interval construction methods was comparable, with the delta method demonstrating 95% coverage plus or minus only a few percent in nearly all settings (Appendix S5 in the **Online Supplementary Document, Figure 3**). The results for the exact and bootstrap method, were similar to the results in the setting with a binary readiness estimate, except that the over- and undercoverage arises in settings with small sample sizes and extreme values of P_{xrf} (binary coverage) only. The exact method and to a lesser extent the bootstrap method resulted in coverage below the nominal 95% level in small samples when P_{xrf} true coverage was less than 10% at any level of readiness or when true coverage was greater than 0.9 and readiness exceeded 0.5 (Appendix S5 in the **Online Supplementary Document, Figure 2**, Panel A, **Figure 4,** Panel A). Coverage probabilities were all close to 95% once both sample sizes reached 500.

Applied example

Figure 5 shows the adjusted coverage estimates and 95% confidence intervals constructed with the exact and delta methods for the nine combinations of coverage and quality measures, as described in the Methods section. Adjusted coverage of ANC in Senegal differed as expected, based on the definitions of coverage and readiness, from a high of 89% using a single ANC visit and facility readiness, such as blood pressure apparatus, to a low of less than 1% for all estimates based on receiving eight or more ANC visits. Confidence intervals are wider with the delta method, although for most estimates, both methods provide largely overlapping intervals. At the national level, all intervals were within the bounds of 0 to 1, although for the region-specific estimates (Appendix S6 in the **Online Supplementary Document**) with smaller sample size, the exact method produced 33 (out of 126) invalid confidence intervals that crossed the 0, 1 bounds. These violations affected the estimates near the boundaries: ANC 1 and blood pressure apparatus on the high end, and all estimates based on ANC 8 and/or appropriate hemoglobin and urine protein diagnostic capacity on the low end. The delta method could not be applied in the 24 cases where the adjust-

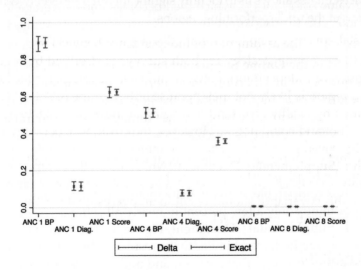

Figure 5. *Adjusted coverage estimates of antenatal care in Senegal with 95% confidence intervals using the delta and exact methods. Coverage is defined as 1, 4, or 8 antenatal care visits (ANC 1, ANC 4, ANC 8 respectively). Readiness is defined based on functional blood pressure apparatus (BP), functional diagnostics (Diag.), or summary score (Score).*

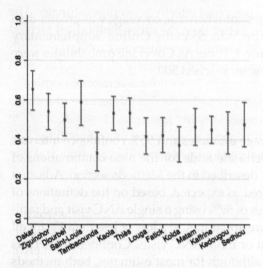

Figure 6. *Adjusted coverage of antenatal care in 14 regions of Senegal with 95% confidence intervals using the delta method. Results are shown for coverage defined as at least 4 antenatal care visits and readiness defined as functional blood pressure apparatus.*

ed coverage estimate was 0 for a particular type of coverage and a given sub-national region. While the exact method confidence intervals are symmetrical, using the logit transformation in the delta method produces asymmetrical intervals to better reflect the bounds of a proportion. In the case of regions with small sample sizes and adjusted coverage estimates near 1, the lower bound could be quite large, for instance adjusted coverage of 1 ANC visit using blood pressure apparatus as the readiness measure is 97.8%, 95% CI = 15.3%-100%.

Calculating confidence and variance in these adjusted coverage estimates enables inference to be drawn on the results. **Figure 6** shows the delta method results for service readiness based on blood pressure apparatus for four ANC visits. Depicting the variance around the point estimates allows us to identify significant differences between regions and to target the underperforming regions.

In this example, the assumption of independence between regions is likely met as the sampling strategy for both surveys is stratified by region. The assumption of independence between adjusted coverage for facility types within a region is likely not met, because although the SPA facility survey is stratified by facility type (and managing authority), the DHS household survey is not and could not be. However, the covariance between the facility-specific coverage estimates within a region is negative (see Appendix S7 in the **Online Supplementary Document**), which makes the covariance between the facility-specific *effective coverage* estimates within region negative as well. Ignoring this covariance should result in an overestimate of variance and a conservative confidence interval.

DISCUSSION

Effective coverage is the product of two quantities with their own sampling error, and as such, is an atypical parameter for variance estimation. In this paper, we evaluated the performance of the exact, delta, and bootstrap methods for constructing confidence intervals around effective coverage estimates. The delta method approach performed better than the other methods: it yielded close to nominal coverage, ie, that 95% confidence intervals captured the truth in 95% of the simulations for a given setting, in nearly all cases. The exact and parametric bootstrap methods resulted in undercoverage of nominally 95% confidence intervals – leading to Type I errors in inference – in settings with small sample sizes or coverage and quality measures close to 0 or 1. The exact method also produced invalid confidence intervals in such settings. The non-parametric bootstrap demonstrated consistent undercoverage and was not analyzed in detail.

We applied the delta and exact methods to calculate adjusted coverage of antenatal care in Senegal, using a sample of women with recent live births from the DHS household survey and a sample of health facilities from the SPA facility audit. Both data sources provide estimates with their own sampling error. Using the delta and exact methods enabled us to incorporate both sources of variance. The results demonstrate that the delta and exact methods can be applied to obtain confidence intervals for complex survey data at sub-national and national levels to support inference around levels and trends in adjusted coverage measures. The delta method was more robust in providing valid results even for small sub-national regions; researchers should be aware that confidence intervals may be quite wide for adjusted coverage estimates near 1.

This work shows that it is feasible to characterize the uncertainty around an effective coverage estimate calculated from separate data sources. Variance estimation should become standard practice if effective coverage estimates are to become part of national and global health monitoring [2,5,33]. The methods outlined here may further be applicable to effective coverage estimation in educational settings, such as the human capacity index developed by the World Bank to capture years of quality-adjusted education as a composite measure of years of schooling and achievement test scores [34,35]. Accurate estimation of variability enables stronger inferences that can inform comparisons and targeted improvement actions. Of the methods considered here, we recommend using the delta method approach – because of its superior performance compared to the exact and bootstrap methods, and since the bootstrap approach outlined in this paper has not yet been adapted for effective coverage estimates based on complex survey designs. In order to facilitate use of these methods, we provide code that can be used by researchers for constructing confidence intervals in a variety of settings, including with complex survey data such as the DHS and SPA.

One limitation of this work is that the simulation studies considered the setting in which the quantities used for effective coverage estimation are computed using simple random samples from the data sources; we note that while we expect the relative performance of the methods to hold for quantities estimated using data from a complex sample, the precise coverage levels may differ to a small extent. A second limitation is that to simplify the variance expressions for the exact and delta methods, any covariance between the facility-level or regional-level effective coverage estimates is ignored. In other words, the facility/region-specific effective coverage estimates are taken to be independent in the derivation of the variance formulas. The assumption is not required for cases with a single geographic area and single facility type (or homogeneous quality measures across observed facility types). In the applied example here, where this covariance is nonzero due to dependence of adjusted coverage estimates across different facility types within each region, it is negative and would reduce the variance if accounted for. Investigating the magnitude of this covariance and modifying the methods to take it into account for increased precision are areas for future research.

Researchers should assess the assumptions of independence between region-specific estimates or facility-specific estimates within a region based on the sampling design of the data sources used and note this limitation as relevant. For example, for estimates based on SPA and DHS data, the assumptions for the current analysis would be the same if we further sub-divided facility types by managing authority [30]. However, the assumptions would not hold if adjusted coverage estimates were computed at a geographic level below that used in the sampling schemes for SPA and DHS.

Defining and quantifying variance for effective coverage estimates underscores the atypical elements of this parameter as a product of two proportions or bounded scales. We identified several areas for further investigation on technical elements of the variance. These include modest overcoverage of delta method confidence intervals in the simulation studies with extreme values of coverage and readiness; the assumption that the sampling distribution of F (formula 14, the logit of effective coverage) is approximately normal may not be met in such extreme cases. Further, the poor performance of the non-parametric bootstrap and the lack of parametric bootstrap estimator available for a product of estimates from complex survey data are gaps that warrant development or refinement of bootstrap methods for this setting.

The methods defined here presume that quantities such as facility readiness are measured without sampling error. Further work is required to adapt the confidence interval construction methods to incorporate error in the estimates of coverage or quality. For instance, estimates of quality for adjusted coverage may be based on a sample of health workers [18], observed patient visits [17], or clinical records [36,37]. Researchers must determine if these within-facility measures provide consistent estimates of readiness at the facility level and, if so, how to capture the within-facility sampling error in composite effective coverage.

While incorporating variance in the sampled estimates of coverage and health system quality is important in accurately reporting effective coverage, the methods described here do not incorporate sources of variability that are not captured in the source data. For example, applications of effective coverage estimation frequently combine population data covering a number of years (ANC for live births in the past 2 years would cover visits for pregnancies beginning up to 33 months before the survey) with health system estimates from a single point in time. A particular strength of the data from Senegal used here is that these surveys were conducted simultaneously, but this is more the exception than the rule in existing population and health system surveys. Confidence interval calculation will not address variance introduced from changes in health system measures over time. These sources of uncertainty should be stated in reporting effective coverage results or incorporated via quantitative bias analysis.

Because measures of crude coverage may obscure the deficits of the health system, assessing effective or adjusted coverage is important in order to recognize both the extent of contact with services, as well as the quality of the services received. Uncertainty estimates that account for the variability in the coverage and quality estimates provide more accurate information for understanding the potential range of quality-adjusted coverage and enabling comparison of these estimates over time and between regions, or countries. Yet, until now, estimates of variance have been largely absent from analysis of effective coverage that combined multiple data sources. This study fills this gap by exploring and comparing three methods for calculating variance. We recommend the delta method as the primary approach for variance calculation, provide Stata code for confidence interval calculation, and outline the assumptions researchers should assess in its application to benefit future research.

Acknowledgments: The authors would like to thank Diane Stoy for editorial assistance and the members of the Countdown to 2030 Coverage Technical Working Group, particularly Lara Vaz and Inácio Crochemore M da Silva, for comments on the draft manuscript.

Disclaimer: This work was prepared while Wenjuan Wang was employed at ICF. The opinions expressed in this article are the author's own and do not reflect the view of the National Institutes of Health, the Department of Health and Human Services, or the United States government.

Funding: This work was supported by a grant of the Bill & Melinda Gates Foundation to the Countdown to 2030 for Women's, Children's and Adolescents' Health, through US Fund for UNICEF (OPP1148933), and by the United States Agency for International Development (USAID) through The DHS Program (#720-OAA-18C-00083).

Author contributions: Conceptualization: HHL, TP. Methodology: TP, SMS. Software: SMS, TP, HHL. Analysis: SMS, WW, LM, HHL. Visualization: SMS, LM, HHL. Writing original draft: SMS, HHL. Review and editing: SMS, TP, WW, LM, HHL.

Competing interests: The authors completed the Unified Competing Interest form at www.icmje.org/coi_disclosure.pdf (available upon request from the corresponding author). Dr Leslie reports grant support from the Bill & Melinda Gates Foundation during the conduct of the study. The authors declare no other conflicts of interest.

Additional material

Online Supplementary Document

Reference

1 United Nations Development Program. Sustainable development goals. Geneva, Switzerland: United Nations, 2015.

2 Kruk ME, Gage A, Arsenault C, Jordan K, Leslie H, Roder-DeWan S, et al. High quality health systems—time for a revolution: Report of the Lancet Global Health Commission on High Quality Health Systems in the SDG Era. Lancet Glob Health. 2018;6:e1196-252. Medline:30196093 doi:10.1016/S2214-109X(18)30386-3

3 Ng M, Fullman N, Dieleman JL, Flaxman AD, Murray CJL, Lim SS. Effective coverage: a metric for monitoring universal health coverage. PLoS Med. 2014;11:e1001730. Medline:25243780 doi:10.1371/journal.pmed.1001730

4 Countdown to 2030 Collaboration. Countdown to 2030: tracking progress towards universal coverage for reproductive, maternal, newborn, and child health. Lancet. 2018;391:1538-48. Medline:29395268 doi:10.1016/S0140-6736(18)30104-1

5 Amouzou A, Leslie HH, Ram M, Fox M, Jiwani S, Requejo J, et al. Advances in the measurement of coverage for RMNCH and nutrition: from Contact to Effective Coverage. BMJ Glob Health. 2019;4 Suppl 4:e001297. Medline:31297252 doi:10.1136/bmjgh-2018-001297

6 Boerma T, AbouZahr C, Evans D, Evans T. Monitoring intervention coverage in the context of universal health coverage. PLoS Med. 2014;11:e1001728. Medline:25243586 doi:10.1371/journal.pmed.1001728

7 Do M, Micah A, Brondi L, Campbell H, Marchant T, Eisele T, et al. Linking household and facility data for better coverage measures in reproductive, maternal, newborn, and child health care: systematic review. J Glob Health. 2016;6:020501. Medline:27606060 doi:10.7189/jogh.06.020501

8 Department of Reproductive Health and Research, Family and Community Health. WHO Antenatal Care Randomized Trial: Manual for the Implementation of the New Model. Geneva, Switzerland: World Health Organization, 2002.

9 United Nations. The Millennium Development Goals Report 2015. New York, New York: United Nations, 2015.

10 World Health Organization. WHO recommendations on antenatal care for a positive pregnancy experience. Geneva, Switzerland: World Health Organization, 2016.

11 Baker U, Okuga M, Waiswa P, Manzi F, Peterson S, Hanson C. Bottlenecks in the implementation of essential screening tests in antenatal care: Syphilis, HIV, and anemia testing in rural Tanzania and Uganda. Int J Gynaecol Obstet. 2015;130:S43-50. Medline:26054252 doi:10.1016/j.ijgo.2015.04.017

12 Baker U, Peterson S, Marchant T, Mbaruku G, Temu S, Manzi F, et al. Identifying implementation bottlenecks for maternal and newborn health interventions in rural

districts of the United Republic of Tanzania. Bull World Health Organ. 2015;93:380-9. Medline:26240459 doi:10.2471/BLT.14.141879

13 Heredia-Pi I, Serván-Mori E, Darney BG, Reyes-Morales H, Lozano R. Measuring the adequacy of antenatal health care: a national cross-sectional study in Mexico. Bull World Health Organ. 2016; 94:452-61. Medline:27274597 doi:10.2471/BLT.15.168302

14 Hodgins S, D'Agostino A. The quality-coverage gap in antenatal care: toward better measurement of effective coverage. Glob Health Sci Pract. 2014;2:173-81. Medline:25276575 doi:10.9745/GHSP-D-13-00176

15 Kanyangarara M, Munos MK, Walker N. Quality of antenatal care service provision in health facilities across sub–Saharan Africa: Evidence from nationally representative health facility assessments. J Glob Health. 2017;7:021101. Medline:29163936 doi:10.7189/jogh.07.021101

16 Kiwanuka Henriksson D, Fredriksson M, Waiswa P, Selling K, Swartling Peterson S. Bottleneck analysis at district level to illustrate gaps within the district health system in Uganda. Glob Health Action. 2017;10:1327256. Medline:28581379 doi:10.1080/16549716.2017.1327256

17 Leslie HH, Malata A, Ndiaye Y, Kruk ME. Effective coverage of primary care services in eight high-mortality countries. BMJ Glob Health. 2017;2:e000424. Medline:29632704 doi:10.1136/bmjgh-2017-000424

18 Marchant T, Tilley-Gyado RD, Tessema T, Singh K, Gautham M, Umar N, et al. Adding content to contacts: Measurement of high quality contacts for maternal and newborn health in Ethiopia, North East Nigeria, and Uttar Pradesh, India. PLoS One. 2015;10:e0126840. Medline:26000829 doi:10.1371/journal.pone.0126840

19 Nguhiu PK, Barasa EW, Chuma J. Determining the effective coverage of maternal and child health services in Kenya, using demographic and health survey data sets: tracking progress towards universal health coverage. Trop Med Int Health. 2017;22:442-53. Medline:28094465 doi:10.1111/tmi.12841

20 World Health Organization. World Bank. Tracking Universal Health Coverage: First Global Monitoring Report. World Health Organization, World Bank, 2015.

21 Colson KE, Zúñiga-Brenes P, Ríos-Zertuche D, Conde-Glez CJ, Gagnier MC, Palmisano E, et al. Comparative estimates of crude and effective coverage of measles immunization in low-resource settings: Findings from Salud Mesoamérica 2015. PLoS One. 2015;10:e0130697. Medline:26136239 doi:10.1371/journal.pone.0130697

22 Aaron GJ, Strutt N, Boateng NA, Guevarra E, Siling K, Norris A, et al. Assessing program coverage of two approaches to distributing a complementary feeding supplement to infants and young children in Ghana. PLoS One. 2016;11:e0162462. Medline:27755554 doi:10.1371/journal.pone.0162462

23 Wang W, Mallick L, Allen C, Pullum T. Effective coverage of facility delivery in Bangladesh, Haiti, Malawi, Nepal, Senegal, and Tanzania. PLoS One. 2019;14:e0217853. Medline:31185020 doi:10.1371/journal.pone.0217853

24 Willey B, Waiswa P, Kajjo D, Munos M, Akuze J, Allen E, et al. Linking data sources for measurement of effective coverage in maternal and newborn health: what do we learn from individual- vs ecological-linking methods? J Glob Health. 2018;8:010601. Medline:29497508 doi:10.7189/jogh.06.0207028.010601

25 Munos MK, Maiga A, Do M, Sika GL, Carter ED, Mosso R, et al. Linking household survey and health facility data for effective coverage measures: a comparison of ecological and individual linking methods using the Multiple Indicator Cluster Survey in Côte d'Ivoire. J Glob Health. 2018;8:020803. Medline:30410743 doi:10.7189/jogh.08.020803

26 Wang W, Mallick L, Allen C, Pullum T. Effective coverage of facility delivery in Bangladesh, Haiti, Malawi, Nepal, Senegal, and Tanzania. Rockville, Maryland: ICF, 2018.

27 Goodman LA. On the Exact Variance of Products. J Am Stat Assoc. 1960;55:708-13. do i:10.1080/01621459.1960.10483369

28 Hogg RV, Craig AT. Introduction to mathematical statistics. 2nd ed. New York: Macmillan Publishing Co., Inc.; 1965.

29 Efron B. Bootstrap methods: Another look at the jackknife. Ann Stat. 1979;7:1-26. doi:10.1214/aos/1176344552

30 Agence Nationale de la Statistique et de la Démographie (ANSD) [Sénégal], ICF International. Sénégal: Enquête Continue sur la Prestation des Services de Soins de Santé (ECPSS) 2014. Rockville, Maryland: Agence Nationale de la Statistique et de la Démographie (ANSD) [Sénégal] and ICF International, 2015.

31 World Health Organization. Service Availability and Readiness Assessment (SARA) Implementation Guide. Geneva, Switzerland: World Health Organization, 2015 September 2015. Report No.: Contract No.: Version 2.2.

32 Lahiri P. On the impact of bootstrap in survey sampling and small-area estimation. Stat Sci. 2003;18:199-210. doi:10.1214/ss/1063994975

33 Lozano R, Soliz P, Gakidou E, Abbott-Klafter J, Feehan DM, Vidal C, et al. Benchmarking of performance of Mexican states with effective coverage. Lancet. 2006;368:1729-41. Medline:17098091 doi:10.1016/S0140-6736(06)69566-4

34 World Bank. World Development Report 2019: The Changing Nature of Work. Washington DC: The World Bank, 2019.

35 World Bank. World Development Report 2018: Learning to Realize Education's Promise. Washington DC: The World Bank, 2018.

36 Chaturvedi S, Upadhyay S, De Costa A, Raven J. Implementation of the partograph in India's JSY cash transfer programme for facility births: a mixed methods study in Madhya Pradesh province. BMJ Open. 2015;5:e006211. Medline:25922094 doi:10.1136/bmjopen-2014-006211

37 Khan ANS, Billah SM, Mannan I, Mannan II, Begum T, Khan MA, et al. A cross-sectional study of partograph utilization as a decision making tool for referral of abnormal labour in primary health care facilities of Bangladesh. PLoS One. 2018;13:e0203617. Medline:30188940 doi:10.1371/journal.pone.0203617

Section 2

Monitoring coverage and quality care

Timing and number of antenatal care contacts in low- and middle-income countries: Analysis in the Countdown to 2030 priority countries

Safia S Jiwani[1], Agbessi Amouzou[1], Liliana Carvajal[2], Doris Chou[3], Youssouf Keita[1], Allisyn C Moran[4], Jennifer Requejo[2], Sanni Yaya[5], Lara ME Vaz[6], Ties Boerma[7]

[1] Department of International Health, Johns Hopkins Bloomberg School of Public Health, Baltimore, Maryland, USA

[2] Data and Analytics Section, Division of Data, Analytics, Planning and Monitoring, UNICEF, New York, New York, USA

[3] Department of Reproductive Health and Research, World Health Organization, Geneva, Switzerland

[4] Department of Maternal, Newborn, Child and Adolescent Health and Aging, World Health Organization, Geneva, Switzerland

[5] School of International Development and Global Studies, University of Ottawa, Ottawa, Ontario, Canada

[6] Department of Global Health, Save the Children US, Washington, District of Columbia, USA

[7] Department of Community Health Sciences, Rady Faculty of Health Sciences, Max Rady College of Medicine, University of Manitoba, Winnipeg, Manitoba, Canada

Background The 2016 World Health Organization (WHO) guidelines for antenatal care (ANC) shift the recommended minimum number of ANC contacts from four to eight, specifying the first contact to occur within the first trimester of pregnancy. We quantify the likelihood of meeting this recommendation in 54 Countdown to 2030 priority countries and identify the characteristics of women being left behind.

Methods Using 54 Demographic and Health Surveys (DHS) and Multiple Indicator Cluster Surveys (MICS) since 2012, we reported the proportion of women with timely ANC initiation and those who received 8-10 contacts by coverage levels of ANC4+ and by Sustainable Development Goal (SDG) regions. We identified demographic, socio-economic and health systems characteristics of timely ANC initiation and achievement of ANC8+. We ran four multiple regression models to quantify the associations between timing of first ANC and the number and content of ANC received.

Results Overall, 49.9% of women with ANC1+ and 44.3% of all women had timely ANC initiation; 11.3% achieved ANC8+ and 11.2% received no ANC. Women with timely ANC initiation had 5.2 (95% confidence interval (CI) = 5.0-5.5) and 4.7 (95%

CI = 4.4-5.0) times higher odds of receiving four and eight ANC contacts, respectively ($P < 0.001$), and were more likely to receive a higher content of ANC than women with delayed ANC initiation. Regionally, women in Central and Southern Asia had the best performance of timely ANC initiation; Latin America and Caribbean had the highest proportion of women achieving ANC8+. Women who did not initiate ANC in the first trimester or did not achieve 8 contacts were generally poor, single women, with low education, living in rural areas, larger households, having short birth intervals, higher parity, and not giving birth in a health facility nor with a skilled attendant.

Conclusions Timely ANC initiation is likely to be a major driving force towards meeting the 2016 WHO guidelines for a positive pregnancy experience.

Antenatal care (ANC) is a platform for the delivery of essential services to prevent pregnancy complications, provide counselling for birth and emergency preparedness [1], and improve health outcomes for children [2]. Timely initiation of antenatal care, defined as the first antenatal care contact occurring within the first trimester of pregnancy, provides an opportunity for early screening of modifiable risk-factors and pre-existing conditions [3].

The 2016 WHO recommendations on antenatal care for a positive pregnancy experience suggest a shift from the focused ANC model with a recommended minimum of four ANC visits (ANC4+) to a more expanded model emphasizing number, timing, and content of contacts. This model suggests a minimum of eight ANC contacts, with the first contact taking place in the first trimester of gestation, followed by two and five contacts in the second and third trimesters, respectively [4]. The expansion from a minimum of four to eight ANC contacts highlights the critical need to further target women who initiate ANC late, who are less likely to achieve the new recommended threshold for a positive pregnancy experience.

The achievement of the formerly recommended ANC4+ has been a priority indicator for monitoring maternal health globally and is used in global initiatives such as the Countdown to 2030 [5], the Ending Preventable Maternal Mortality (EPMM) [6], and the Global Strategy for women's, children's and adolescents' health [7]. Conversely, timely first ANC has not been widely reported on, but has been shown to be associated with the total number of ANC contacts achieved and the content of care received [8,9]. Although the global coverage of one skilled ANC contact remains high at 86% [10], a substantially lower proportion of pregnant women initiate ANC during the first trimester [3]. Reasons associated with delayed ANC initiation include financial constraints, distance to health facilities, cultural and religious beliefs around disclosure of pregnancy status, gender norms, lack of awareness of pregnancy signs and antenatal care schedules, pregnancy wantedness, perceptions on the need to start ANC early, and quality of care received [1,11-19].

Nevertheless, little evidence exists on the status of timely ANC initiation on a global scale. A recent study by Moller et al. suggested that the coverage of timely ANC initiation in 2013 was at 24.0% in low-income countries compared to 81.9% in high-income countries [3]. However, further analyses are needed to characterize the profile of women who initiate ANC late, the likelihood of receiving basic components, the standing of countries that are falling behind, and what it will take to improve the timing and number of routine ANC contacts to meet the revised WHO guidelines. Our study addresses these questions in the 81 Countdown to 2030 priority countries [5], accounting for 95% of global maternal deaths and 90% of deaths among children under-five globally. Specifically, we aim to (1) quantify the timing of ANC initiation and its variation according to overall levels of ANC contacts, (2) compare the profile of women who initiated ANC during the first trimester to that of women who delayed the first visit until the second or third trimester, (3) quantify the association between timely ANC initiation and a) the number of ANC contacts received and b) the content of ANC care received, (4) estimate the proportion of women who achieve ANC8+ contacts and compare their profile to that of women with 1-7 ANC contacts.

METHODS

Data

We searched the latest available Demographic and Health Surveys (DHS) and Multiple Indicator Cluster Surveys (MICS) of all 81 Countdown to 2030 priority countries since 2012 for data on timing of first ANC contact and number of ANC contacts achieved. The year 2012 cut off was used to ensure that estimates produced are recent across the countries included in the analysis. 54 countries with latest DHS or MICS surveys carried out between 2012 and May 2018 were included in the analysis: 45 DHS and 9 MICS surveys. We restricted the analysis to the last live birth in the two years preceding the survey reported by women aged 15-49 interviewed during the survey. The 54 surveys include a total of 290 783 such births, ranging from 932 in Guyana to 91 614 in India, with available data on timing and number of ANC (Table S1 in the **Online Supplementary Document**).

The DHS and MICS are nationally-representative household surveys implemented in over 90 low- and middle-income countries that provide data on health and population indicators. The surveys include samples of women of reproductive age, generally 15-49 years, who are asked about information on their pregnancies in the last five years or their last pregnancy. Both sets of surveys collect information on ANC, including the timing of first ANC contact through the question "how many weeks/months pregnant were you when you first received antenatal care for this pregnancy?". Information on the total number of ANC contacts and selected basic ANC components received are also collected.

Main variables

Our main outcome of interest, timing of antenatal care, was the self-reported gestational age at which the respondent had her first ANC contact during her pregnancy for the index child. We recoded the gestational age variable collected in DHS and MICS into months from one to nine and defined timely initiation of ANC as a first contact occurring within the first trimester. Additional variables included the total number of ANC contacts received and the content of care received, both captured as self-reported variables in DHS and MICS. The number of ANC contacts was further grouped into ANC4+ and ANC8+.

To assess receipt of basic ANC components during ANC contacts, we relied on the limited information collected in the surveys on content of care received at least once during ANC, available across both type of surveys. These include blood pressure measurement, urine test, blood test, and HIV testing and receipt of result. Although they do not capture the full set of components required during ANC, together they provide an indication of whether some basic services could be recalled by the women. We created a content of antenatal care variable as a categorical score (0, 1, 2+), defined as the number of components reported to have been received at least once during pregnancy, out of the total of four components considered.

Statistical analysis

We carried out statistical analyses using individual country data sets as well as a pooled data set of all countries. For the latter, the analysis was weighted by the inverse proportion of sampled births contributed by each country in the pooled data set, to adjust for the size of the sample of each country data set. We analyzed the timing of ANC for the total sample as well as by three groups of countries based on their coverage of ANC4+ (<50%, 50%-75%, and 75% or more), and by regions based on the Sustainable Development Goals regional grouping.

Within our second aim, we assessed the characteristics of women with timely ANC initiation by comparing their demographic, socio-economic and health systems factors to that of women with delayed ANC initiation, stratifying by ANC4+ coverage levels. We then fit a multiple logit regression of timely ANC initiation on these factors to uncover the significant predictors.

We quantified the associations between timing of first ANC and the number as well as the content of ANC by running four different multiple regression analyses. First, we fitted a linear regression of ANC contacts on gestational age at the first ANC in months; then we ran separate logistic regressions of ANC4+ and ANC8+ on timely ANC initiation. Lastly, we ran a multinomial ordered logistic regression of the ANC content score, treated as a categorical dependent outcome, on timely ANC initiation, treated as a binary independent variable. All regression models were adjusted for country as well as demographic and socio-economic factors.

Finally, we estimated the coverage of 0, 1-3, 4-7, 8-10 ANC contacts by countries' ANC4+ coverage levels and geographic regions, and characterized women who received 8-10 contacts compared to those who had 1-7 contacts by demographic, socio-economic and health systems variables.

All analyses were conducted with Stata 15 [20] and took into account the sampling weights and the complex survey design. Figures were generated on Microsoft Excel 2016 (Microsoft Inc, Seattle WA, USA) and Stata 15 (Stata Corp, College Station, TX, USA).

Ethical consideration

DHS and MICS are publicly available de-identified data. Ethical approval was not needed for analysis of the data. Ethical approval for data collection was the responsibility of the institutions that collected the data.

RESULTS

Coverage and distribution of timely ANC initiation

Across the 54 countries, the median gestational age at first ANC was three months, with an interquartile range between three and five months. Overall, 11.2% of women had no ANC during pregnancy. Half of women (49.9%) with at least one ANC contact initiated it within the first trimester of pregnancy; 43.3% and 6.8% delayed until the second and third trimesters respectively (**Table 1**). The coverage of timely ANC initiation varied by level of ANC4+ coverage and by geographic region. In countries where less than 50% of women achieved ANC4+, representing over half of the pooled data, 37.9% of women had timely ANC initiation, compared to 61.3% in countries where 75% or more women achieved ANC4+. By geographic region, Central and Southern Asia, and Latin America and the Caribbean recorded the largest proportions of timely ANC initiation among women with at least one ANC contact (69.1% and 68.1%, respectively), compared to 40.8% in Sub-Saharan Africa. **Figure 1** shows considerable disparities in timing of ANC across countries, and Figure

Table 1. *Distribution of timely ANC initiation by level of ANC4+ coverage and region among women with at least one ANC**

	MEDIAN GESTATIONAL AGE AT FIRST ANC CONTACT (IQR)	TIMING OF FIRST ANC AMONG WOMEN WITH ANC₁₊ (N = 243 967)		
		1st trimester (n = 128 495), % (95% CI)	2nd trimester (n = 99 168), % (95% CI)	3rd trimester (n = 16 304), % (95% CI)
Country groups by ANC4+ coverage level:				
1 (<50%)	3 (3-5)	37.9 (37.2-38.7)	51.3 (50.7-52.0)	10.7 (10.3-11.1)
2 (50%-74%)	4 (3-5)	47.2 (46.5-47.9)	45.9 (45.2-46.5)	6.9 (6.6-7.2)
3 (75% +)	3 (2-4)	61.3 (60.6-62.1)	34.9 (34.2-35.6)	3.8 (3.6-4.1)
SDG region:				
Central and Southern Asia[†]	3 (2-4)	69.1 (67.9-70.3)	25.0 (24.0-26.1)	5.9 (5.4-6.4)
Eastern and South-Eastern Asia[‡]	3 (2-4)	63.5 (62.3-64.7)	31.4 (30.3-32.5)	5.1 (4.6-5.6)
Latin America and the Caribbean [§‡]	3 (2-4)	68.1 (66.9-69.2)	28.5 (27.4-29.7)	3.4 (3.0-3.8)
Northern Africa and Western Asia[ǁ]	3 (2-5)	54.6 (53.0-56.1)	32.9 (31.6-34.3)	12.5 (11.6-13.5)
Sub-Saharan Africa[¶]	4 (3-5)	40.8 (40.3-41.4)	51.7 (51.2-52.2)	7.5 (7.3-7.7)
Total among women with ANC1⁺:				
Pooled	3 (3-5)	49.9 (49.5-50.4)	43.3 (42.9-43.7)	6.8 (6.6-7.0)

ANC – antenatal care, IQR – interquartile range, CI – confidence interval, SDG – Sustainable Development Goal
*Note: % are row percentages, n unweighted.
[†]Central and Southern Asia: Afghanistan, India, Kyrgyz Republic, Nepal, Pakistan, Tajikistan, Turkmenistan.
[‡]Eastern and South-Eastern Asia: Cambodia, Indonesia, Lao People's Democratic Republic, Myanmar, Philippines, Timor Leste.
[§]Latin America and the Caribbean: Dominican Republic, Guatemala, Guyana, Haiti, Honduras, Paraguay.
North Africa and Western Asia: Sudan, Yemen.
[¶]Sub-Saharan Africa: Angola, Burundi, Comoros, Eswatini, Ethiopia, Kenya, Lesotho, Malawi, Namibia, Rwanda, Uganda, Tanzania, Zambia, Zimbabwe, Benin, Cameroon, Chad, Congo, Cote D'Ivoire, Democratic Republic of Congo, Gabon, Gambia, Ghana, Guinea, Guinea-Bissau, Liberia, Mali, Mauritania, Niger, Nigeria, Senegal, Sierra Leone, Togo.

S1 in the **Online Supplementary Document** maps out the coverage of timely ANC initiation in countries included in the analysis. However, the top 10 highest performers in terms of timely ANC initiation include countries from all regions, suggesting that achieving such performance by countries that are still behind is possible, and may not be tied to regional characteristics. Turkmenistan is the best performer in timely ANC initiation (89.6%), with almost universal use of antenatal care services. Conversely, Nigeria is the lowest performer (12.9%) with a substantial proportion of women with no ANC.

Who are the women who initiate ANC on time?

Table 2 presents socio-economic and demographic characteristics of women with timely ANC initiation, as well as health systems characteristics as reported by them, stratified by the three groups of countries based on ANC4+ coverage. Overall, compared to women with delayed ANC initiation, a significantly higher proportion of women with timely ANC initiation resided in urban areas (39.5% vs 30.7%), had secondary or higher education (48.7% vs 33.2%), lived in smaller households of one to four members (28.2% vs 24.6%), and belonged to the highest wealth quintile (21.0% vs 13.1%). They were at their first child

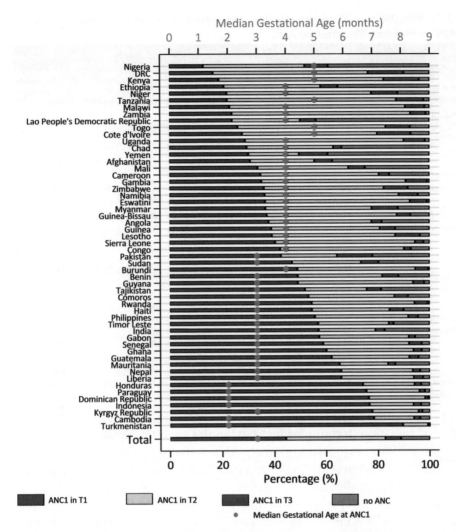

Figure 1. *Distribution of births by gestation trimester at first antenatal care (ANC) contact, and median gestation months by country.*

(30.4% vs 24.4%) or a child with birth order between 2 and 4 (51.7% vs 48.6%), had birth with preceding interval of five years or more (16.1% vs 13.5%), and were married (75.2% vs 71.1%). In terms of health systems characteristics, a larger proportion of women with timely ANC initiation received antenatal care in a hospital (35.5% vs 28.7%) or from the formal private sector at least once, had an institutional birth (77.4% vs 66.3%), attended the formal public sector for delivery (65.0% vs 57.4%), and had a skilled attendant at birth (82.4% vs 70.1%). Additionally, a higher proportion of women with timely ANC initiation across the three groups received at least two or more components of ANC content (88.8% vs 79.6%).

Table 2. *Demographic, socio-economic and health systems characteristics of women with timely ANC initiation among those with at least one ANC*

ANC4+ COVERAGE LEVEL	COUNTRY GROUP 1 (<50% ANC4+) (N = 133 064)[†]		COUNTRY GROUP 2 (50% -74% ANC4+) (N = 61 749)[†]		COUNTRY GROUP 3 (≥75% ANC4+) (N = 49 154)[†]		POOLED (N = 243 967)[†]	
Women's characteristics	1st trimester	2nd/3rd trimester	1st trimester	2nd/3rd trimester	1st trimester	2nd/3rd trimester	1st trimester	2nd/3rd trimester
Demographic and socio-economic								
Median age at birth (IQR)	24 (21-28)	25 (21-29)	26 (21-31)	26 (21-31)	26 (21-31)	25 (21-31)	25 (21-29)	25 (21-30)
Residence:								
Urban	33.2*	22.5	39.0*	30.7	42.8	40.3	39.5*	30.7
Rural	66.8*	77.5	61.0*	69.3	57.2	59.7	60.5*	69.3
Education:								
No education	35.9*	43.3	28.5*	31.0	11.0*	18.2	22.0*	31.2
Primary	33.1*	37.3	31.8*	39.7	26.0	27.6	29.4*	35.5
Secondary/Higher	31.0*	19.4	39.6*	29.2	63.0*	54.3	48.7*	33.2
Number of HH members:								
1-4	27.8*	24.3	26.3*	24.1	29.9*	25.5	28.2*	24.6
5-6	28.2	28.5	28.1	28.5	32.2*	28.8	29.9*	28.6
7+	43.9*	47.2	45.7	47.4	37.9*	45.7	41.9*	46.9
Sex of head of household:								
Male	87.2	86.2	76.6*	78.5	75.7*	71.0	78.3	78.9
Female	12.8	13.8	23.4*	21.5	24.3*	29.0	21.7	21.1
Wealth index:								
Q1 (poorest)	15.8*	21.8	17.9*	23.2	21.0*	26.3	18.9*	23.6
Q2	17.1*	22.3	18.7*	23.1	20.7*	22.9	19.3*	22.8
Q3	19.3*	20.9	20.2	21.6	20.8	20.4	20.3	21.1
Q4	21.4	20.2	21.3*	19.2	19.7	18.7	20.6*	19.4
Q5 (richest)	26.4*	14.8	21.9*	12.9	17.9*	11.6	21.0*	13.1
Birth order:								
1	28.9*	21.6	29.2*	24.2	32.1*	27.9	30.4*	24.4
2-4	49.2*	46.5	49.6	48.4	54.5*	51.4	51.7*	48.6
5+	21.9*	31.8	21.2*	27.4	13.5*	20.7	17.9*	27.0
Preceding birth interval:								
First child	29.0*	21.7	29.4*	24.3	32.2*	28.0	30.6*	24.5
≤2 y	15.1*	17.0	13.4	14.4	12.6*	14.2	13.4*	15.2
3-4 y	42.9*	49.4	43.6*	48.8	35.7*	41.2	39.9*	46.9
5+ years	13.0	11.9	13.5	12.5	19.6*	16.7	16.1*	13.5
Marital status:								
Single	3.1*	4.9	4.4*	7.5	7.3*	14.9	5.4*	8.7
Married	84.6*	79.0	82.4*	75.0	65.2*	56.6	75.2*	71.1
Other	12.3*	16.1	13.2*	17.5	27.5	28.5	19.4	20.1
Health systems								
Place of ANC:								
Hospital	37.8*	27.6	33.9*	27.4	35.4*	31.9	35.5*	28.7
Health Center	44.0	46.2	36.8*	44.5	27.4*	34.1	34.3*	42.3
Other formal	15.7*	24.4	26.3	25.4	36.1*	31.9	28.2	26.8
Other informal	2.4*	1.8	3.0	2.7	1.2*	2.0	2.1	2.2
Sector of place for ANC:								
Public formal	76.7*	84.4	85.8*	88.3	81.4*	88.4	81.8*	86.9
Private formal	20.8*	13.8	11.2*	8.9	17.3*	9.6	16.1*	10.9
Other/ informal	2.5*	1.8	3.0	2.7	1.3*	2.0	2.1	2.2
ANC content (4 components):								
None	6.1*	11.6	2.8*	4.7	1.0*	2.4	2.6*	6.3
1 component	14.1*	21.4	7.1*	12.4	7.2	8.0	8.5*	14.1
2+ components	79.8*	67.0	90.2*	82.9	91.8*	89.7	88.8*	79.6

Table 2. *Continued*

ANC4+ COVERAGE LEVEL	Country Group 1 (<50% ANC4+) (N = 133 064)[†]		Country Group 2 (50% -74% ANC4+) (N = 61 749)[†]		Country Group 3 (≥75% ANC4+) (N = 49 154)[†]		Pooled (N = 243 967)[†]	
Women's characteristics	1st trimester	2nd/3rd trimester	1st trimester	2nd/3rd trimester	1st trimester	2nd/3rd trimester	1st trimester	2nd/3rd trimester
Place of delivery:								
Health facility	73.4*	61.0	71.6*	63.9	83.8*	75.8	77.4*	66.3
Home	25.8*	37.9	26.5*	34.6	15.2*	23.1	21.3*	32.5
Other	0.9	1.1	1.9	1.5	1.0	1.0	1.3	1.2
Sector of place of delivery:								
Public formal	58.7*	52.3	62.5*	55.4	69.8*	66.0	65.0*	57.4
Private formal	14.7*	8.7	9.8	8.8	14.4*	10.0	12.8*	9.1
Other informal	26.7*	39.0	27.7*	35.8	15.8*	24.1	22.2*	33.5
Attendant at birth:								
Unskilled	23.0*	36.0	21.7*	31.8	12.0*	20.0	17.6*	29.9
Skilled	77.0*	64.0	78.3*	68.2	88.0*	80.0	82.4*	70.1

ANC – antenatal care, IQR – interquartile range, CI – confidence interval, HH – household members
*Non-overlapping 95% confidence intervals between women who initiated ANC in the first trimester and those who initiated ANC in the second or third trimester, for that characteristic.
[†]Note: n is unweighted.

Similar patterns were observed in each ANC4+ coverage group, with few exceptions. In the low ANC4+ coverage group, a larger proportion of women with timely ANC initiation attended ANC in the informal sector (2.4% vs 1.8%); this was not observed in the middle and high ANC4+ coverage groups. In the medium ANC4+ coverage group, there was a higher proportion of female-headed households (23.4% vs 21.5%). Both in the low and medium coverage groups, a higher proportion of women with timely ANC initiation lived in urban areas compared to those with delayed ANC initiation.

Across all three country groups, predictors of timely ANC initiation included education and wealth, married status, smaller household size and parity (Table S2 in the **Online Supplementary Document**).

Association between timing of ANC initiation and number and content of ANC received

Table 3 presents the results of the multiple regression models assessing the association between timing of ANC initiation and the number of contacts as well as the content of ANC received. Overall, women with timely ANC initiation are significantly more likely to achieve four and eight or more ANC contacts (aOR = 5.24 with 95% CI = 5.04-5.45 and 4.66 with 95% CI = 4.35-4.99 respectively, $P < 0.001$), and to receive higher ANC content during pregnancy (aOR = 1.66 with 95% CI = 1.59-1.73, $P < 0.001$). Furthermore, every one-month delay in ANC initiation reduces the total number of ANC contacts reached by 0.62 ($\beta = -0.62$ with 95% CI = -0.63, -0.61 and $P < 0.001$).

Table 3. *Positive associations between timely ANC initiation and number and content of ANC received*

Model	Independent variable	Dependent variable	Crude β[†] (95% CI)	Adjusted β[‡] (95% CI)	Crude OR[†] (95% CI)	Adjusted OR[‡] (95% CI)
1	Gestational age (months) at first ANC contact	Number of ANC contacts	-0.66* (-0.67, -0.65)	-0.62* (-0.63, -0.61)		
2	Timely ANC (1st trimester)	ANC4+			5.82* (5.60, 6.04)	5.24* (5.04, 5.45)
3	Timely ANC (1st trimester)	ANC8+			5.32* (4.98, 5.68)	4.66* (4.35, 4.99)
4	Timely ANC (1st trimester)	ANC content			2.02* (1.94-2.11)	1.66* (1.59-1.73)

ANC – antenatal care, CI – confidence interval
*Coefficients significant at $P < 0.001$.
[†]Adjusted by country.
[‡]Adjusted by country, demographic and socio-economic variables.

Figure 2 gives the breakdown of monthly gestational age at first ANC and the number of ANC contacts achieved. From the figure it can be seen that reaching eight contacts or more requires starting ANC during the first month of gestation. While 58% of women who initiated ANC in the first month achieved eight or more contacts, only 24% of those who initiated ANC in the second month achieved this number. The percentage dropped to 9% for those who initiated ANC in the third month.

Further assessment showed that over half of women who initiated ANC in the first trimester received each of the four ANC interventions (urine test, blood test, blood pressure, HIV test and received results). The proportion dropped to about 40% when ANC was initiated in the second trimester, and to 5% in the third trimester (Figure S2 in the **Online Supplementary Document**).

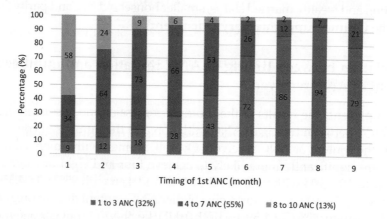

Figure 2. *Number of antenatal care (ANC) contacts by timing of ANC initiation, among women with at least one ANC (n = 243 967).*

Who are the women who receive a minimum of eight ANC contacts?

Table 4 shows the distribution of the number of ANC contacts by coverage of ANC4+ and by SDG region. Overall, 11.2% of women reported not having received any ANC during pregnancy, whereas 28.3% received 1-3 contacts, 49.3% received 4-7 contacts, and 11.3% achieved eight or more contacts during pregnancy.

Coverage of ANC8+ varies by country groups of ANC4+ coverage. ANC8+ coverage is at 3.8% in countries where ANC4+ is <50% and 6.2% when ANC4+ is between 50% and 75%; in countries with ANC4+ coverage above 75%, one in four women achieved eight or more contacts. Regionally, Latin America and the Caribbean had the highest coverage of ANC8+ at 34.3% compared to the lowest in Sub-Saharan Africa at 6.1%; it also had the highest ANC utilization, with 4.3% of women reporting no ANC (**Table 4**).

Table 4. *Distribution of number of ANC contact coverage by ANC4+ country groups and regions among all women**

	NUMBER OF ANC CONTACTS (N = 290 783)			
	No ANC (n = 46 816)	1-3 ANC (n = 95 425)	4-7 ANC (n = 120 578)	8-10 ANC (n = 27 964)
Country group by ANC4+ level:				
	% (95% CI)	% (95% CI)	% (95% CI)	% (95% CI)
1 (<50%)	21.6 (20.9-22.4)	40.1 (39.4-40.8)	34.5 (33.8-35.2)	3.8 (3.6-4.0)
2 (50%-74%)	9.2 (8.8-9.7)	31.9 (31.3-32.5)	52.7 (52.0-53.4)	6.2 (5.8-6.5)
3 (≥75%)	4.1 (3.8-4.4)	13.9 (13.4-14.3)	58.5 (57.8-59.2)	23.5 (22.9-24.2)
SDG regions:				
Central and Southern Asia[†]	14.9 (13.9-16.0)	27.5 (26.4-28.7)	44.2 (42.9-45.6)	13.3 (12.5-14.1)
Eastern and South-Eastern Asia[‡]	14.0 (13.2-14.8)	17.6 (16.7-18.5)	46.8 (45.7-47.9)	21.7 (20.8-22.7)
Latin America and the Caribbean[§]	4.3 (3.9-4.8)	12.1 (11.3-13.0)	49.3 (48.0-50.5)	34.3 (33.0-35.7)
Northern Africa and Western Asia[ǀ]	29.6 (28.1-31.0)	32.8 (31.6-34.1)	29.9 (28.5-31.2)	7.8 (7.1-8.5)
Sub-Saharan Africa[¶]	9.7 (9.3-10.1)	32.3 (31.8-32.8)	51.9 (51.4-52.5)	6.1 (5.8-6.3)
Total:				
Pooled	**11.2 (10.9-11.5)**	**28.3 (27.9-28.7)**	**49.3 (48.8-49.7)**	**11.3 (11.0-11.6)**

ANC – antenatal care, IQR – interquartile range, CI – confidence interval

*Note: % are row percentages, n unweighted.

[†]Central and Southern Asia: Afghanistan, India, Kyrgyz Republic, Nepal, Pakistan, Tajikistan, Turkmenistan.

[‡]Eastern and South-Eastern Asia: Cambodia, Indonesia, Lao People's Democratic Republic, Myanmar, Philippines, Timor Leste.

[§]Latin America and the Caribbean: Dominican Republic, Guatemala, Guyana, Haiti, Honduras, Paraguay.

[ǀ]North Africa and Western Asia: Sudan, Yemen.

[¶]Sub-Saharan Africa: Angola, Burundi, Comoros, Eswatini, Ethiopia, Kenya, Lesotho, Malawi, Namibia, Rwanda, Uganda, Tanzania, Zambia, Zimbabwe, Benin, Cameroon, Chad, Congo, Cote D'Ivoire, Democratic Republic of Congo, Gabon, Gambia, Ghana, Guinea, Guinea-Bissau, Liberia, Mali, Mauritania, Niger, Nigeria, Senegal, Sierra Leone, Togo.

Figure 3 illustrates the distribution of the number of ANC contacts achieved by country, depicting large variations in ANC8+ ranging from 0% in Rwanda to 53.6% in the Dominican Republic.

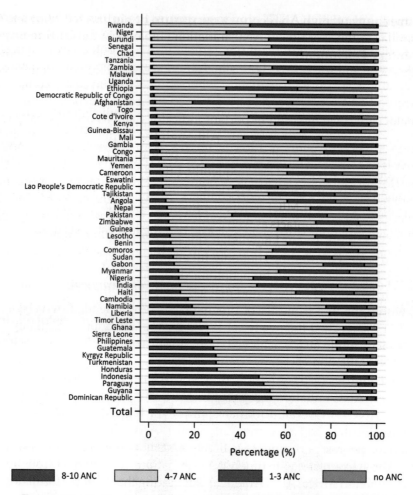

Figure 3. *Distribution of number of antenatal care (ANC) contacts achieved by country.*

The characteristics of women achieving a minimum of eight contacts (Table S3 in the **Online Supplementary Document**) were similar to those with timely ANC initiation. In all three country groups categorized by ANC4+ coverage levels, a significantly larger proportion of women receiving 8-10 ANC compared to 1-7 ANC were urban residents, had secondary or higher education, belonged to the top two wealth quintiles, had a parity of one, were married, received ANC from a hospital or in the private formal sector, and received at least two components of ANC content. Additionally, a larger proportion of these women had an institutional delivery and a skilled attendant at birth. Conversely, in the low ANC4+ coverage group, a higher proportion of women achieving ANC8+ attended ANC in the informal sector; this was not observed in the medium and high ANC4+ coverage groups. Predictors of ANC8+ were also similar to those of timely ANC initiation (Table S4 in the **Online Supplementary Document**).

DISCUSSION

Antenatal care coverage is an important indicator that has been globally reported on to assess maternal health. Although the evidence on number of ANC contacts is readily available, countries' performance in terms of timing of ANC initiation is reported less frequently. Effective promotion of antenatal care and a positive pregnancy experience among women in low- and middle-income countries (LMIC) requires a good understanding of the timing and patterns of ANC contacts as well as the characteristics of women who are likely to fall behind. To our knowledge, this has not been previously studied at a global scale. Our findings not only fill an important gap in the scientific literature, but serve as a call for action for decision-makers. Our analysis of 290 783 births from 54 LMIC found that less than half of the women initiated ANC within the first trimester of pregnancy as recommended by WHO. A total of 11.2% reached the newly set WHO recommendation of a minimum of 8 contacts, while 60.6% achieved at least four contacts. The coverage of timely ANC initiation varied by countries' coverage level of ANC4+: in high coverage countries (≥75% ANC4+), 61.3% of women with at least one ANC had a timely ANC initiation compared to 37.9% in countries with low coverage (<50% ANC4+). Overall, Turkmenistan had the highest coverage of timely ANC initiation (89.6% of all women) and highest ANC utilization, and Nigeria depicted the poorest performance in timely ANC initiation (12.9% of all women). The top 10 countries with timely ANC initiation are scattered throughout three continents (Africa, Asia, America), suggesting that their performance is achievable by other countries. These are also countries that have made progress in reducing inequalities in coverage. For example, Turkmenistan has achieved almost inexistent inequalities, and is the Countdown to 2030 priority country with the highest composite coverage index (CCI), indicating high coverage of reproductive maternal and newborn health services across the continuum of care; whereas Nigeria has recorded some of the largest socio-economic inequalities and lowest CCI [5]. Regionally, Central and Southern Asia followed by Latin America and the Caribbean had the best performance of timely ANC initiation. Conversely, Sub-Saharan Africa is falling behind.

The achievement of 8-10 ANC contacts followed a similar pattern, with a quarter of women in high ANC4+ coverage countries receiving at least eight contacts, compared to 3.8% in low ANC4+ countries. This suggests that for countries where coverage of ANC4+ is below 75%, the large majority among countries in this study, achieving high coverage levels of ANC8+ will be a very steep climb. This is less so for countries with ANC4+ above 75%. Latin America and the Caribbean outperformed the other regions, with the Dominican Republic having the overall highest proportion of women reaching 8-10 ANC (53.6%), compared to Sub-Saharan Africa where Rwanda was the lowest performer with no women reaching eight contacts. Further analyses are needed to understand the specific case of Rwanda, where health systems reforms have led to improvement of maternal health outcomes [21]; however our data suggested that despite having 54.4% of women with timely initiation, none reported achieving eight contacts. The previous recommendation of ANC4+, which was adopted as a policy in all countries and implemented in routine ANC may have affected the overall report of ANC contacts by pregnant women. A cross-sectional study assessing factors of poor ANC utilization in Rwanda indicated that older age, single status, large households and lack of social support were associated with poor ANC utilization of two or less contacts during pregnancy [22].

Other studies have also documented the high ANC performance in Latin America and Caribbean [23]: although this region has the largest income inequalities globally, with varying ANC performance across countries, programs targeting the most vulnerable such as performance-based contracts and conditional-cash transfer schemes have been successful at promoting ANC utilization in recent years [23,24].

Our analyses suggested a strong, independent effect of timing of ANC initiation on the number of contacts, as well as the content of care received. Women with timely ANC initiation had 5.2 (95% CI = 5.0-5.5) and 4.7 (95% CI = 4.4-5.0) times higher odds of achieving at least four and eight ANC contacts respectively, and 1.7 (95% CI = 1.6-1.7) times higher odds of receiving a higher ANC content overall. Further analysis by month of gestation showed that even among women who initiated ANC in a timely manner, those who started in the first month were more likely to report a minimum of 8 contacts. It is unclear whether the ANC contact schedule of these women was consistent with the recommended schedule by WHO, given that DHS and MICS surveys only capture the timing of the first contact.

Women with low education and wealth status, living in larger households, having short birth intervals and higher parity were less likely to begin antenatal care in a timely manner and achieve eight contacts. Strategies to increase ANC contacts must target these women. Our findings were consistent with other studies [1,24-28]: one of them examined coverage and timing of ANC among the poor in Mesoamerican countries and showed that education, parity and marital status were factors predicting timely ANC initiation [24]. Similarly, Gupta et al. looked at utilization of antenatal care in Tanzania between 1990 and 2010 and found that urban residence, lower birth order and ANC initiation before four months of gestation were associated with utilization of at least four antenatal care visits [1].

A number of studies have explored reasons for no or delayed ANC initiation, and have included factors such as financial constraints, distance from the health facility, lack of knowledge about the recommended timing of ANC initiation, and socio-cultural factors such as lack of permission from spouse, late disclosure of pregnancy status, pregnancy wantedness [12-16,18,19,29,30]. These factors, in addition to the characteristics studied here of women falling behind in terms of timing and number of ANC, should be taken into consideration for specific ANC targeting and programmatic purposes.

The newly set WHO recommendation of a minimum of eight ANC contacts, with higher frequency of contacts almost every two weeks in the third trimester, did not identify effective strategies to overcome the challenges and obstacles mentioned above. Our analyses suggest that achieving such target will be a steep climb for most countries, who will need to put in place policy and programs that tackle both service demand and the strengthening of the health system, including the delivery mechanisms of services, infrastructures and commodities, and the monitoring of these services. It will not be surprising if these countries are hesitant to adopt the new recommendations, or worse, implement it only in areas that already have higher ANC coverage, thus further increasing equity gaps. Supportive programmatic measures and resources will be needed to avoid disturbance to already fragile systems. Implementation research can help identify effective and scalable strategies.

Quality of antenatal care content is difficult to measure in household surveys, given that existing questions in these surveys are limited and focus on receipt of components reported by the mother, and don't assess the quality per say of services received. Benova and colleagues examined the coverage and content of ANC in 10 LMIC, and indicated the need for improved measurement of ANC quality: their results suggested that content of care was poor even among women with adequate number and timing of ANC [31]. Our study suggested that women initiating ANC in a timely manner were more likely to receive a higher number of preventive screening components as part of ANC. Mixed methods and qualitative studies are crucial to get a better picture of the quality of services received, including respectful care and satisfaction. Furthermore, linking household surveys to health facility assessments will also be an important step towards improved coverage measurement.

Our analysis has several limitations. The variables on timing, number and content of antenatal care were based on self-reported events, which are subject to recall-bias. This was also the case for the assessment of gestational age based on self-report by the mother. Limiting the analysis to the last live birth in the two years preceding the survey may have reduced this bias. Coverage estimates rely heavily on self-reported data obtained from household surveys, yet little is known on the validity of these estimates, particularly in LMIC settings. A validation study in Southwestern China in 2011 found that self-reported coverage of routine ANC interventions had overall poor validity, and timing of 1st ANC prior to 12 weeks of gestation had a large population-level bias [32]. In our study, the recall of timing of first ANC was recorded in months rather than weeks, and there could have been a bias leading to overestimation of the proportion of women receiving ANC1 in the first trimester. In addition, there may have been social desirability bias in the number of ANC reported, although this was less likely to be an issue for ANC8+ given it has not yet been adopted widely. We excluded women who reported more than ten contacts; although we considered these to be over-reporting cases, they could also describe ANC behaviors for very sick mothers or those with high obstetric risks. However, the proportion was low (3.8% of the pooled data set) and would have negligible effects on our results. We assessed content of ANC using four components reported to have been received at least once during ANC. These were not comprehensive nor the most important components of antenatal care, but rather the ones most commonly reported in DHS and MICS surveys. Moreover, no information was available on the contacts at which these components were received.

CONCLUSIONS

In conclusion, our findings from 54 priority Countdown countries show that timely ANC initiation is a major driving force for meeting the 2016 WHO antenatal care guidelines for a positive pregnancy experience. This achievement appears feasible in short to medium term in countries where coverage of ANC4+ is very high. For most countries, achieving high coverage levels of ANC8+ will require strong policy change and implementation, and dedicated resources to reaching vulnerable and poor populations that are still not accessing the services. In order to ensure that no woman is left behind, programs and policies promoting antenatal care services ought to bridge the gap and focus on the most vulnerable women whose needs in antenatal care aren't being met. Strong implementation research is needed to learn about effective strategies.

Acknowledgements: The authors thank the women who participated in the DHS and MICS surveys, Gulam Muhammed Kibria for initial assistance in the analysis and the Countdown Coverage Technical Working Group for inputs in earlier versions of the analysis.

Funding: Bill & Melinda Gates Foundation. The funder had no role in the writing of this manuscript.

Authorship contributions: *AA conceived the paper and developed the analysis plan. SSJ carried out the analysis and wrote the initial draft. All authors reviewed earlier drafts and approved the final manuscript.*

Competing interests: *The authors completed the Unified Competing Interest form at www.icmje.org/coi_disclosure.pdf (available upon request from the corresponding author), and declare no conflicts of interest.*

Additional material
Online Supplementary Document

References

1 Gupta S, Yamada G, Mpembeni R, Frumence G, Callaghan-Koru JA, Stevenson R, et al. Factors associated with four or more antenatal care visits and its decline among pregnant women in Tanzania between 1999 and 2010. PLoS One. 2014;9:e101893. Medline:25036291 doi:10.1371/journal.pone.0101893

2 Kuhnt J, Vollmer S. Antenatal care services and its implications for vital and health outcomes of children: evidence from 193 surveys in 69 low-income and middle-income countries. BMJ Open. 2017;7:e017122. Medline:29146636 doi:10.1136/bmjopen-2017-017122

3 Moller AB, Petzold M, Chou D, Say L. Early antenatal care visit: a systematic analysis of regional and global levels and trends of coverage from 1990 to 2013. Lancet Glob Health. 2017;5:e977-83. doi:10.1016/S2214-109X(17)30325-X. Medline:28911763

4 World Health Organization. WHO Recommendation on Antenatal care for positive pregnancy experience. WHO Recomm Antenatal care Posit pregnancy Exp. 2016; Available: http://apps.who.int/iris/bitstream/10665/250796/1/9789241549912-eng.pdf. Accessed: 22 February 2019.

5 United Nations, Children's Fund (UNICEF) and the World Health Organization (WHO). Tracking Progress towards Universal Coverage for Reproductive, Newborn and Child Health: The 2017 Report. 2017. Available: http://countdown2030.org/pdf/Countdown-2030-complete-with-profiles.pdf. Accessed: 22 February 2019.

6 World Health Organization. Strategies toward ending preventable maternal mortality (EPMM). 2015;6736:1–4. Available: http://who.int/reproductivehealth/topics/maternal_perinatal/epmm/en/. Accessed: 22 February 2019.

7 WHO, UNAIDS, UNFPA, UNICEF, UNWomen, The World Bank Group. Survive, Thrive, Transform. Global Strategy for Women's, Children's and Adolescents' Health: 2018 report on progress towards 2030 targets. 2018. Available: http://www.who.int/life-course/partners/global-strategy/gswcah-monitoring-report-2018.pdf?ua=1. Accessed: 22 February 2019.

8 Saad–Haddad G, DeJong J, Terreri N, Restrepo–Méndez MC, Perin J, Vaz L, et al. Patterns and determinants of antenatal care utilization: analysis of national survey data in seven countdown countries. J Glob Health. 2016;6:010404. Medline:27231540 doi:10.7189/jogh.06.010404

9 Agha S, Tappis H. The timing of antenatal care initiation and the content of care in Sindh, Pakistan. BMC Pregnancy Childbirth. 2016;16:190. Medline:27460042 doi:10.1186/s12884-016-0979-8

10 UNICEF. Antenatal Care. 2018. Available: https://data.unicef.org/topic/maternal-health/antenatal-care/. Accessed: 22 February 2019.

11 Aduloju OP, Akintayo AA, Ade-Ojo IP, Awoleke JO, Aduloju T, Ogundare OR. Gestational age at initiation of antenatal care in a tertiary hospital, Southwestern Nigeria. Niger J Clin Pract. 2016;19:772-7. Medline:27811450 doi:10.4103/1119-3077.181398

12 Ifenne DI, Utoo BT. Gestational age at booking for antenatal care in a tertiary health facility in north-central, Nigeria. Niger Med J. 2012;53:236-9. Medline:23661885 doi:10.4103/0300-1652.107602

13 Oladokun A, Oladokun RE, Morhason-Bello I, Bello AF, Adedokun B. Proximate predictors of early antenatal registration among Nigerian pregnant women. Ann Afr Med. 2010;9:222-5. Medline:20935421 doi:10.4103/1596-3519.70959

14 Onoh R, Umeora OUJ, Agwu UM, Ezegwui HU, Ezeonu PO, Onyebuchi AK. Pattern and Determinants of Antenatal Booking at Abakaliki Southeast Nigeria. Ann Med Health Sci Res. 2012;2:169-75. Medline:23439716 doi:10.4103/2141-9248.105666

15 Belayneh T, Adefris M, Andargie G. Previous early antenatal service utilization improves timely booking: Cross-sectional study at university of Gondar Hospital, northwest Ethiopia. J Pregnancy. 2014;2014. Medline:25101176 doi:10.1155/2014/132494

16 Exavery A, Kanté AM, Hingora A, Mbaruku G, Pemba S, Phillips JF. How mistimed and unwanted pregnancies affect timing of antenatal care initiation in three districts in Tanzania. BMC Pregnancy Childbirth. 2013;13:35. Medline:23388110 doi:10.1186/1471-2393-13-35

17 Kaswa R, Rupesinghe GFD, Longo-Mbenza B. Exploring the pregnant women's perspective of late booking of antenatal care services at Mbekweni Health Centre in Eastern Cape, South Africa. Afr J Prim Health Care Fam Med. 2018;10:e1-9. Medline:30035599 doi:10.4102/phcfm.v10i1.1300

18 Ochako R, Gichuhi W. Pregnancy wantedness, frequency and timing of antenatal care visit among women of childbearing age in Kenya. Reprod Health. 2016;13:51 Medline:27142068 doi:10.1186/s12978-016-0168-2

19 Gulema H, Berhane Y. Timing of First Antenatal Care Visit and its Associated factors among pregnant women attending public health facilities in Addis Ababa, Ethiopia. Ethiop J Health Sci. 2017;27:139-46. Medline:28579709 doi:10.4314/ejhs.v27i2.6

20 StataCorp. Stata Statistical Software: Release 15. College Station TSL. Stata Statistical Software. 2017.

21 Haver J, Brieger W, Zoungrana J, Ansari N, Kagoma J. Experiences engaging community health workers to provide maternal and newborn health services: Implementation of four programs. Int J Gynaecol Obstet. 2015;130:S32-9. Medline:26115855 doi:10.1016/j.ijgo.2015.03.006

22 Rurangirwa AA, Mogren I, Nyirazinyoye L, Ntaganira JKG. Determinants of Poor Utilization of Antenatal Care Services among Recently Delivered Women in Rwanda: A Population Based Study. BMC Pregnancy Chiildbirth. 2017;17:142. Medline:28506265 doi:10.1186/s12884-017-1328-2

23 Amo-adjei J, Aduo-adjei K, Opoku-nyamah C, Izugbara C. Analysis of socioeconomic differences in the quality of antenatal services in low and middle-income countries (LMICs). PLoS One. 2018;13:1-12.

24 Dansereau E, McNellan CR, Gagnier MC, Desai SS, Haakenstad A, Johanns CK, et al. Coverage and timing of antenatal care among poor women in 6 Mesoamerican countries. BMC Pregnancy Childbirth. 2016;16:234. Medline:27542909 doi:10.1186/s12884-016-1018-5

25 Paudel YR, Jha T, Mehata S. Timing of first antenatal care (ANC) and inequalities in early initiation of ANC in Nepal. Front Public Health. 2017;5:242. Medline:28955707 doi:10.3389/fpubh.2017.00242

26 Moore N, Blouin B, Razuri H, Casapia M, Gyorkos TW. Determinants of first trimester attendance at antenatal care clinics in the Amazon region of Peru: A case-control study. PLoS One. 2017;12:e0171136. Medline:28207749 doi:10.1371/journal.pone.0171136

27 Aliyu AA, Dahiru T. Predictors of delayed Antenatal Care (ANC) visits in Nigeria: secondary analysis of 2013 Nigeria Demographic and Health Survey (NDHS). Pan Afr Med J. 2017;26:124. Medline:28533847 doi:10.11604/pamj.2017.26.124.9861

28 Kuuire VZ, Kangmennaang J, Atuoye KN, Antabe R, Boamah SA, Vercillo S, et al. Timing and utilisation of antenatal care service in Nigeria and Malawi. Glob Public Health. 2017;12:711-27. Medline:28441926 doi:10.1080/17441692.2017.1316413

29 Kien VD, Van Minh H, Giang KB, Dao A, Weinehall L, Eriksson M, et al. Socioeconomic inequalities in self-reported chronic non-communicable diseases in urban Hanoi, Vietnam. Glob Public Health. 2017;12:1522-37. Medline:26727691 doi:10.1080/17441692.2015.1123282

30 Gidey G, Hailu B, Nigus K, Hailu T, Gher W, Gerensea H. Timing of first focused antenatal care booking and associated factors among pregnant mothers who attend antenatal care in Central Zone, Tigray, Ethiopia. BMC Res Notes. 2017;10:608. Medline:29162155 doi:10.1186/s13104-017-2938-5

31 Benova L, Tunçalp Ö, Moran AC, Campbell OMR. Not just a number: examining coverage and content of antenatal care in low-income and middle-income countries. BMJ Glob Health. 2018;3:e000779. Medline:29662698 doi:10.1136/bmjgh-2018-000779

32 Liu L, Li M, Yang L, Ju L, Tan B, Walker N, et al. Measuring coverage in MNCH: A Validation study linking population survey derived coverage to maternal, newborn, and child health care records in rural China. PLoS One. 2013;8:e60762. Medline:23667429 doi:10.1371/journal.pone.0060762

Evaluating coverage of maternal syphilis screening and treatment within antenatal care to guide service improvements for prevention of congenital syphilis in Countdown 2030 Countries

Shivika Trivedi[1], Melanie Taylor[2,3], Mary L Kamb[3], Doris Chou[2]

[1] CDC Foundation, Atlanta, Georgia, USA
[2] World Health Organization, Geneva, Switzerland
[3] Centers for Disease Control and Prevention (CDC), Atlanta, Georgia, USA

Background Countdown to 2030 (CD2030) tracks progress in the 81 countries that account for more than 90% of under-five child deaths and 95% of maternal deaths in the world. In 2017, CD2030 identified syphilis screening and treatment during antenatal care (ANC) as priority indicators for monitoring.

Methods Country-reported data in the UNAIDS Global AIDS Monitoring System (GAM) system were used to evaluate four key syphilis indicators from CD2030 countries: (1) maternal syphilis screening and (2) treatment coverage during ANC, (3) syphilis seroprevalence among ANC attendees, and (4) national congenital syphilis (CS) case rates. A cascade analysis for CD2030 countries with coverage data for the number of women attending at least 4 antenatal care visits (ANC4), syphilis testing, seroprevalence and treatment was performed to estimate the number of CS cases that were attributable to missed opportunities for syphilis screening and treatment during antenatal care.

Results Of 81 countries, 52 (64%) reported one or more values for CS indicators into the GAM system during 2016-2017; only 53 (65%) had maternal syphilis testing coverage, 49 (60%) had screening positivity, and 41 (51%) had treatment coverage. CS case rates were reported by 13 (16%) countries. During 2016-2017, four countries reported syphilis screening and treatment coverage of ≥95% consistent with World Health Organization (WHO) targets. Sufficient data were available for 40 (49%) of countries to construct a cascade for data years 2016 and 2017. Syphilis screening and treatment service gaps within ANC4 resulted in an estimated total of 103 648 adverse birth outcomes with 41 858 of these occurring as stillbirths among women attending ANC4 (n = 31 914 408). Women not in ANC4 (n = 25 619 784) contributed an additional 67 348 estimated adverse birth outcomes with 27 198 of these occurring as stillbirths for a total of 69 056 preventable stillbirths attributable to syphilis in these 40 countries.

Conclusion These data and findings can serve as an initial baseline evaluation of antenatal syphilis surveillance and service coverage and can be used to guide improvement of delivery and monitoring of syphilis screening and treatment in ANC for these priority countries.

Syphilis is a leading cause of adverse pregnancy outcomes including stillbirth and neonatal death. In 2016, WHO estimated there were 988 000 maternal syphilis infections worldwide resulting in 355 000 adverse pregnancy outcomes, of which over half were stillbirths or neonatal deaths [1,2]. Both screening and treatment for syphilis during pregnancy remain sub-optimal in low- and middle-income countries despite diagnosis and prevention of maternal-to-child transmission (MTCT) of syphilis being feasible, inexpensive and cost-effective [3]. In 2007, WHO and partners launched a global initiative to eliminate congenital syphilis based on the pillars of 1) sustained political commitment and advocacy, 2) access to and quality of maternal and newborn health services; 3) universal syphilis screening for all pregnant women and treatment of women testing positive and their partners; and 4) adequate surveillance, monitoring and evaluation [4]. In 2008, ANC syphilis testing coverage, prevalence, treatment coverage, and congenital syphilis (CS) rate were added as indicators for country monitoring and reporting to the UNAIDS Global AIDS Monitoring (GAM) system [5] and are publicly reported in the WHO Global Health Observatory (GHO) [6]. This was followed by the WHO launch of the *Global Guidance on Criteria and Processes for Validation of Elimination of Mother-to-Child Transmission of HIV and Syphilis* in 2014. The targets countries need to achieve for elimination of MTCT of syphilis are 1) at least 95% of pregnant women attend antenatal care (ANC); 2) at least 95% of pregnant women in ANC receive syphilis screening; and 3) at least 95% of syphilis seropositive pregnant women receive adequate treatment [7].

Countdown to 2030 (CD2030) is a partnership among academic institutions, UN agencies, governments and other civil society members that provides independent analyses that aim to accelerate the achievement of the Sustainable Development Goals for ending preventable maternal, newborn and child deaths [8]. Its efforts are focused on 81 priority countries that account for more than 95% of maternal, and 90% of under-five, child deaths in the world. Moreover, CD2030 aims to utilize regional networks to build the capacity of countries to use evidence-based interventions to shape national plans and policies [9]. In 2018, CD2030 selected prevention of MTCT of syphilis as one of their initiatives and added the WHO ANC syphilis testing and treatment indicators to those which each *Countdown* country should monitor.

We aimed to evaluate current maternal and congenital syphilis surveillance systems in the 81 CD2030 countries through examination of two country-reported syphilis service coverage indicators: 1) percentage of pregnant women tested for syphilis and 2) percentage of seropositive pregnant women who were treated for syphilis and coverage of attendance of at least 4 antenatal care visits (ANC4). The aims of this analysis are to: describe coverage of these services in CD2030 countries towards the 95% targets required for WHO validation of CS elimination; highlight gaps in antenatal surveillance that may reflect service gaps and estimate the number of CS-associated stillbirths and other adverse birth outcomes due to service gaps within ANC and among women not attending ANC in CD2030 countries. Country use of the GAM reporting system for reporting these indicators is also described. Given the burden of maternal and neonatal disease in these countries, progress achieved in preventing CS in CD2030 countries will help to drive progress towards achieving the goals of the Global Strategy for Women, Children, and Adolescent Health [10] and the Sustainable Development Goals [8] related to improvements in maternal and newborn health.

METHODS

We utilized the Global AIDS Monitoring (GAM) surveillance system, which collates country-reported HIV/AIDS outcome and coverage indicators. Since 2008, GAM has included four key syphilis indicators: (i) maternal syphilis screening coverage and (ii) maternal syphilis treatment coverage during ANC, (iii) syphilis seroprevalence among ANC attendees, and (iv) national reported CS case rates, data which are publicly available in GHO [6]. We focused our analysis on the 81 countries prioritized by CD2030. The most recent data reported by countries during the 2-year interval from 2016 and 2017 were utilized to describe the percentage of pregnant women who were screened and treated for syphilis by country over this time period.

We applied a CS prevention cascade to estimate the number of CS cases that could be attributed to a service gap at each level of ANC service (ie, ANC attendance, syphilis testing, and treatment) similar to methods used to estimate the global burden of CS [1]. This estimate utilized those CD2030 countries with numerator and denominator data for ANC4, syphilis screening, diagnosis and treatment for data years 2016 or 2017. United Nations estimates of live births were combined with a global estimate of stillbirth to generate an estimate of total number of pregnancies for each country [11-14]. ANC was defined as attendance at a minimum of four ANC visits (ANC4) with data obtained from the WHO Department of Reproductive Health and Research ANC4+ Global Database March 2019 [15].This database contains data that are extracted from publicly available sources. Aggregate data reported from 2016-2017 among included countries were utilized to estimate the sum of women in ANC4 who were tested and not tested, the seroprevalence of syphilis in women attending ANC4, and the sum of ANC4 women who were seropositive that were treated and not treated. The number of women who were in ANC4 and not tested and the number of women not in ANC4 were multiplied by the reported maternal syphilis seroprevalence from GAM and added to the women that tested positive in ANC4 but were not treated to estimate the number of WHO-defined congenital syphilis cases attributable to a missed opportunity in ANC4 [13,16]. To estimate burden of active, transmissible syphilis, a standard syphilis test type correction factor was applied to adjust for syphilis test positivity that could be due to previously treated syphilis consistent with global CS estimation methods [1,17]. Lastly, we applied the previous estimate that untreated cases of maternal syphilis among women in ANC4 and not in ANC4, incurred a 52% risk of adverse birth outcomes (ABOs) and a 21% risk of stillbirth, to estimate the total number of ABOs and stillbirths that were due to CS and could have been avoided with maternal syphilis screening and treatment in 2016-2017 amongst these CD2030 countries [1,13, 16].

We used the WHO case definition of congenital syphilis pertaining to infants born to pregnant women with untreated syphilis as follows [7]:

"The WHO global surveillance case definition for congenital syphilis includes A live birth or fetal death at >20 weeks of gestation or >500 g (including stillbirth) born to a woman with positive syphilis serology and without adequate syphilis treatment."

We assumed reported treatment coverage reflected the WHO definition of adequate treatment to prevent congenital syphilis defined as at least one injection of 2.4 million units of benzathine penicillin given at least 30 days prior to delivery. We also evaluated the reported syphilis diagnostic test types used, with a focus on the uptake of rapid syphilis testing over the two-year period 2016-2017. For evaluation of indicators and diagnostic test type, those countries not reporting any data for 2016 to 2017, or only reporting data prior to 2016, were considered "Missing/Unknown." Microsoft Excel (Microsoft Inc, Seattle, WA, USA) was used for all calculations with results confirmed in SPSS V. 21 (IBM Inc, Armonk, NY, USA).

RESULTS

Of 81 CD2030 countries, 52 (64%) reported one or more values for CS indicators into the GAM system during 2016-2017. Data on maternal syphilis testing coverage was provided by 53 (65%), screening positivity was reported by 49 (60%), treatment coverage was reported by 41 (51%) and syphilis test type was reported by 53 (65%) CD2030 countries. CS case rates were only reported by

13 (16%) CD2030 countries (**Table 1**). Of the 81 CD2030 countries, 40 (49%) reported data for all three indicators related to coverage of services (syphilis testing, test positivity, and treatment of seropositive women) during 2016 and 2017. Reported screening and treatment coverage is summarized in **Table 2**.

Importantly, many countries reporting high treatment coverage reported very low syphilis screening coverage in ANC. Of 28 countries reporting ≥75% treatment coverage, 13 (43%) had <50% coverage for testing and an additional four (14%) had moderate (50%-74%) testing coverage. ANC4 coverage notwithstanding, four CD2030 countries (Bolivia, Burkina Faso, Eritrea, and Tajikistan) met the WHO targets of 95% coverage for both syphilis testing and treatment.

Analysis of the 40 CD2030 countries with data for ANC4, syphilis testing, seroprevalence and treatment was performed to build a CS prevention cascade and estimate the number of CS cases that were attributable to each service delivery gap (N = 59 784 822 pregnant women). (**Figure 1**, Table S1 in the **Online Supplementary Document**). Of 31 914 408 (53%) pregnant women receiving at least four ANC visits in these 40 countries 8 441 392 (26%) were tested for syphilis, while 23 473 016 (74%) pregnant women were in ANC4 but not tested. Based on reported maternal syphilis seroprevalence and testing and treatment coverage, an estimated 199 323 women attended ANC4 with active syphilis but were either not tested, or tested but not treated (WHO-defined CS cases). As previously estimated, 52% of untreated cases of maternal syphilis are estimated to result in ABOs including stillbirths [13,16]. Applying these estimates, the ANC4 service gaps above resulted in a total of 103 648 ABOs with 41 858 of these occurring as stillbirths among women attending ANC4 in the 40 *Countdown* countries with complete data for years 2016 or 2017. Women in the 40 countries that did not attend ANC4 (n = 27 870 414) contributed to the CS burden with an additional 129 516 WHO-defined CS cases with 67 348 estimated ABOs of which 27 198 of were stillbirths (**Figure 1**). In total, 170 996 ABOs were estimated with 69 056 occurring as stillbirths in these 40 countries. The remaining 41 *Countdown* countries (81-40 = 41) did not have data available for this analysis.

During 2016 and 2017, 53 (65%) *Countdown* countries reported the type(s) of syphilis diagnostic tests used for the two-year period in ANC clinics. Of these, 17 (32%) reported use of rapid treponemal-based syphilis tests; 13 (24.5%) reported use of non-treponemal diagnostic tests, such as rapid plasmin reagin (RPR) or venereal disease research laboratory (VDRL) tests, and 23 (43%) reported use of non-treponemal diagnostic tests followed by confirmatory treponemal testing (using *Treponema pallidum* particle agglutination (TPPA) or *Treponema pallidum* haemagglutination (TPHA) assay (**Table 1**).

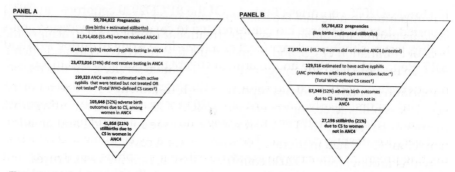

Figure 1. *Estimated congenital syphilis cases associated with missed opportunities for testing and treatment. Panel A. Receipt of Antenatal Care, at least four visits (ANC4). *Test type correction factor applied to percent testing positive and ANC women untested but assumed positive based on prevalence of tested proportion. Panel B. No receipt of ANC. *The same test-type correction factor applied for this proportion of women not attending ANC4 as was applied for those in ANC4. Country-reported maternal syphilis prevalence of women in ANC applied to this calculation (GAM). †The WHO global surveillance case definition for congenital syphilis is A live birth or fetal death at >20 weeks of gestation or >500 g (including stillbirth) born to a woman with positive syphilis serology and without adequate syphilis treatment" [6].*

DISCUSSION

Only half of these 81 *Countdown* countries entered data on syphilis testing and treatment coverage into the UNAIDS GAM system in 2016 or 2017. For many countries, reported ANC syphilis services require scale-up to achieve elimination of maternal-to-child-transmission (EMTCT) by 2030. Using a pre-existing surveillance system, we were able to identify 4 countries that have reported reaching the WHO syphilis service coverage targets for validation of elimination of vertical transmission of syphilis for both testing and treatment of maternal syphilis in 2016-2017. Using a cascade-type analysis, we identified opportunities to improve syphilis testing and treatment coverage that would prevent a large number of preventable ABOs and stillbirths. These analyses demonstrate opportunities for antenatal syphilis surveillance and service improvements as part of congenital syphilis elimination e

By utilizing the UNAIDS GAM system, our data can serve as an evaluation of the current state of coverage of antenatal syphilis surveillance indicators as reported by these 81 priority CD2030 countries. These data allow CD2030 to specifically tailor their congenital syphilis prevention and elimination efforts. Rather than creating a new surveillance system, efforts can be centered on improving reporting and analysis of data reported to UNAIDS GAM, and evaluating reporting and coverage trends over time, as well as surveillance gaps. For this to happen, more CD2030 countries could be supported to report ANC syphilis indicator data to GAM, and those that are now reporting could do so more completely and consistently [5].

It is important to note that the collective targets for ANC coverage, antenatal syphilis testing and antenatal syphilis treatment must be met to achieve the goal of elimination of CS, and women must first have access to, and attend, ANC in order to take advantage of these preventive services. For this reason, reported coverage of each indicator must be interpreted in the context of the other indicators. Nearly, one-third of CD2030 countries (25, 30.9%) reported >75% maternal syphilis treatment coverage, however, many of these countries had very low testing coverage. These countries may be doing a good job at treating pregnant women who are seropositive for syphilis, but they are not doing a good job at screening this population, and thus likely have not seen improvements in CS rates.

As the targets for elimination of CS are predicated on women accessing ANC, the cascade analysis of missed opportunities for prevention demonstrates how service gaps at each level contribute to the total missed opportunities for intervention and CS rate reduction. Using the GAM data for 2016-2017, we were able to estimate the ABOs and stillbirths that are due to missed opportunities within and outside of ANC, data which can be used to support surveillance and service improvements. Moreover, it is important to note that this estimate likely substantially underestimates the number of ABOs and stillbirths attributable to limited syphilis testing and treatment coverage in the CD2030 countries as our cascade analysis was limited to only 40 of 81 CD2030 countries with complete data for each indicator. It is plausible that even with high coverage of syphilis testing, treatment rates may be lower, even in countries that have prioritized efforts to eliminate congenital syphilis, due to shortages of benzathine penicillin during this same time period. Of note, 29 out of 41 countries with shortages in benzathine penicillin between 2014 and 2016 were also CD2030 countries which may explain lower treatment coverage for some [18]. Lastly, it is possible that by virtue of collecting and reporting on these data, these CD2030 countries may in fact, represent the highest coverage for these indicators, which would mean our results grossly underestimate the reality that exists in the remaining CD2030 countries.

The methods used for estimation of CS cases, ABOs and stillbirths in this analysis were similar to those used for global estimation of CS [1]. This analysis differs from that of the recent global CS estimation in that the data input for ANC coverage here was ANC4 whereas ANC1 (at least one ANC visit) was used for the 2016 global CS estimates. The use of ANC4 reflects the WHO modification of the minimum number of ANC visits to 8 contacts in order to achieve effective care during pregnancy, which is now the ANC coverage indicator monitored for CD2030 countries [19]. Data sources for live births were different. Modelling methods used for global estimates of maternal syphilis prevalence were not used here. We assumed reported treatment was adequate

Table 1. *Syphilis screening, positivity, and treatment coverage for 81 Countdown countries 2016-2017**

COUNTRY	SYPHILIS TEST TYPE	WHO REGION	% ANC SCREENING	YEAR % SCREENING	% POSITIVE	YEAR % POSITIVITY	% TREAT	YEAR % TREAT	CS RATE**	YEAR CS RATE
Afghanistan	non-treponemal (RPR,VDRL)/treponemal (rapid tests, TPPA)	Eastern Mediterranean	14.3	2017	0.3	2017	100.0	2017		
Algeria	not reported	Africa								–
Angola	not reported	Africa								
Azerbaijan	not reported	Europe								–
Bangladesh	patients positive on both: non-treponemal/treponemal	South East Asia	72.3	2017	0.0	2017	100.0	2017		–
Benin	non-treponemal (RPR,VDRL) treponemal (rapid tests, TPPA)	Africa	3.1	2017	0.4	2017	100.0	2017		–
Bhutan	not reported	South East Asia								
Bolivia (Plurinational State of)	patients positive on both: non-treponemal/treponemal	Americas	96.0	2017	0.9	2017	100.0	2017		–
Botswana	non-treponemal (RPR,VDRL)	Africa								–
Burkina Faso	non-treponemal (RPR,VDRL) treponemal (rapid tests, TPPA)	Africa	100.0	2016	0.7	2016	100.0	2017	669	2017
Burundi	not reported	Africa								
Cambodia	treponemal (rapid tests, TPPA)	Western Pacific	62.9	2017	0.0	2017	83.9	2017		–
Cameroon	Not reported	Africa								–
Central African Republic	non-treponemal (RPR,VDRL) patients positive on both	Africa	56.1	2017	4.7	2017	97.4	2017		–
Chad	Not reported	Africa								–
Comoros	Not reported	Africa								–
Congo	non-treponemal (RPR,VDRL)	Africa	10.7	2016	0.6	2016				–
Côte d'Ivoire	treponemal (rapid tests, TPPA)	Africa								–
Democratic People's Republic of Korea	not reported	South East Asia								
Democratic Republic of the Congo	non-treponemal (RPR,VDRL) treponemal (rapid tests, TPPA) patients positive on both	Africa								–
Djibouti	not reported	Eastern Mediterranean								–
Dominican Republic	non-treponemal (RPR,VDRL)	Americas	42.2	2017	1.6	2017	54.1	2017		
Equatorial Guinea	not reported	Africa								
Eritrea	treponemal (rapid tests, TPPA)	Africa	97.2	2017	1.1	2017	100.0	2017		–
Ethiopia	not reported	Africa	44.6	2017	1.1	2017	100.0	2017		–

Table 1. Continued

Country	Syphilis test type	WHO region	% ANC screening	Year % screening	% positive	Year % positivity	% treat	Year % treat	CS rate**	Year CS rate
Gabon	non-treponemal (RPR, VDRL)	treponemal (rapid tests, TPPA)	Africa	31.1	2017	1.8	2017	100.0	2017	–	–
Gambia	not reported	Africa					–			–	–
Ghana	non-treponemal (RPR, VDRL)	treponemal (rapid tests, TPPA)	patients positive on both	Africa	44.6	2017	3.0	2017	91.0	2017	–	–
Guatemala	non-treponemal (RPR, VDRL)	treponemal (rapid tests, TPPA)	patients positive on both	Americas	37.1	2017	0.1	2017	47.6	2017	9.2	2017
Guinea	treponemal (rapid tests, TPPA)	Africa	4.8	2017	5.4	2017	100.0	–	–	–
Guinea-Bissau	not reported	Africa								–	–
Guyana	not reported	Americas									
Haiti	treponemal (rapid tests, TPPA)	Americas	92.5	2016	2.8	2016	89.8	2017	–	–
Honduras	non-treponemal (RPR, VDRL)	treponemal (rapid tests, TPPA)	patients positive on both	Americas	69.0	2017	0.2	2017			89.5	2017
India	non-treponemal (RPR, VDRL)	South East Asia	19.8	2017	0.1	2017	47.6	2017	–	–
Indonesia	patients positive on both: non-treponemal/treponemal	South East Asia	1.7	2017	3.2	2017	30.1	2016	1.2	2016
Iraq	not reported	Eastern Mediterranean						–		–
Jamaica	treponemal (rapid tests, TPPA)	Americas	90.0	2016	1.5	2016	70.9	2016	22.8	2016
Kenya	treponemal (rapid tests, TPPA)	Africa	85.7	2017	1.4	2017		–		–
Kyrgyzstan	patients positive on both: non-treponemal/treponemal	Europe	89.4	2017	0.0	2017	100.0	2017	3.2	2017
Lao People's Democratic Republic	not reported	Western Pacific	–		0.8	2009		–		–

Table 2. *Reported performance coverage of antenatal care (ANC) syphilis screening and treatment among Countdown countries (N = 81)*

ANC Syphilis Service Indicator Coverage	95% Coverage*, N (%)	75%–94% Coverage, N (%)	50%–74% Coverage, N (%)	<50% Coverage, N (%)	Data not reported
Syphilis screening	9 (11)	10 (12)	6 (7)	27 (33)	28 (35)
Syphilis treatment†	21 (26)	8 (10)	8 (10)	4 (5)	40 (49)

*WHO target for validation of ending mother-to-child transmission.
†Treatment coverage among those found to be syphilis test positive

for CS prevention and did not estimate residual CS cases occurring due to inadequate or late treatment. Thus, the recently reported 2016 WHO estimates of CS that include these countries cannot be compared to estimates presented here. We readily acknowledge that some countries may collect ANC syphilis screening and treatment coverage but not report into the GAM system. Considering the countries that do utilize GAM, further analyses are needed to definitively identify and address the underlying circumstances to explain high treatment coverage rates in the face of low coverage of testing. For a myriad of reasons, many women do not access ANC. Within ANC, syphilis screening may not be offered due to limited or no testing capacity or it may be offered but at an additional cost. Stock-outs of syphilis test kits and reagents are common, and the need to present to an off-site laboratory for testing may be an additional hurdle. Women may be lost to follow up for treatment after diagnosis of syphilis is made for several reasons. This may include cases where women need to return to a laboratory to obtain results, require outside treatment referrals, have additional costs to receive treatment. Countries may face penicillin shortages resulting in no treatment or providers may use alternative regimens which are not recommended or lack effectiveness data for prevention of CS [18]. Lastly, even those women who are screened and appropriately treated for syphilis remain at risk for re-infection if their partners are not appropriately treated.

Through evaluation of diagnostic test type, it is possible to highlight the use and benefits of rapid syphilis testing in low- and middle-income countries. Among countries reporting test type, approximately one-third (32%) use rapid syphilis tests during ANC. Rapid syphilis testing has the advantage of providing same day results with the opportunity to treat at the time of diagnosis. Utilization of rapid syphilis testing could allow countries to both increase the number of pregnant females screened, while also increasing their treatment coverage within ANC settings where service coverage can be evaluated and monitored. Two rapid dual HIV/syphilis test kits have now received WHO pre-qualification [20] Use of these test kits can result in immediate scale up of syphilis screening alongside that of HIV with the option of same visit treatment for women testing positive for syphilis [21].

These data and this analysis have limitations. Data reporting into the GAM system were inconsistent over the years, some data were implausible, and there are numerous CD2030 countries that did not provide any data into this system. Additional data sources for maternal syphilis screening and treatment of pregnant women may be available but not included in the UNAIDS GAM reporting. It is difficult to know if only the surveillance system is lacking in these countries, or if the coverage of these indicators is also lacking. Same day testing and treatment through the use of point-of-care rapid syphilis tests among women attending only one ANC visit is possible and thus our results could be overestimates for countries where this service is in place. Our analysis of these data are purely descriptive in nature.

These 81 CD2030 countries account for more than 95% of maternal and 90% of under-five child mortality in the world [22]. As a result, uptake of effective syphilis interventions in pregnancy by these countries is well placed to decrease overall levels of preventable, adverse maternal and neonatal outcomes, and eliminate congenital syphilis. To our knowledge this study represents the first evaluation of antenatal syphilis screening and treatment coverage in the 81 CD2030 countries using data reported into the UNAIDS GAM system, as well as the first estimate of ABOs and stillbirths attributable to these service gaps in CD2030 countries where data are available. We encourage countries to improve ANC syphilis screening and treatment coverage and to prioritize the use of the UNAIDS GAM system to capture and monitor progress towards EMTCT [7]. Information on the downstream effects of missed opportunities to screen and treat women for syphilis during ANC provide a rich source of evidence for scale up [23,24].

Acknowledgments: *The authors would like to acknowledge Ann-Beth Moller for her assistance in data collection.*

Disclaimer: *The findings and conclusions in this report are those of the authors and do not necessarily represent the official position of the World Health Organization, or the U.S. Centers for Disease Control and Prevention.*

Funding: *The project was funded by the World Health Organization, Department of Reproductive Health and Research, and Human Reproduction Program STI program and furthermore supported by a cooperative agreement from the US Centers for Disease Control and Prevention in support of strengthening STI surveillance and eliminating congenital syphilis.*

Authorship contributions: *ST, MK, DC, and MT conceived the analysis, MT and DC collected data, ST and MT performed the data analysis, ST, MK, DC, and MT wrote the manuscript. All authors contributed to the final version of the manuscript.*

Competing interests: *The authors completed the ICMJE Unified Competing Interest form (available upon request from the corresponding author), and declare no conflicts of interest.*

Additional material
Online Supplementary Document

References
1 Korenromp EL, Rowley J, Alonso M, Brito de Mello M, Wijesooriya NS, Mahiané SG, et al. Global burden of maternal and congenital syphilis and associated adverse birth outcomes – estimates for 2016 and progress since 2012. PLoS One. 2019;14:e1002473.
2 World Health Organization. Report on global sexually transmitted infection surveillance. Geneva: WHO; 2018.

3 Kahn JG, Jiwani A, Gomez GB, Hawkes SJ, Chesson HW, Broutet N, et al. The cost and cost-effectiveness of scaling up screening and treatment of syphilis in pregnancy: a model. PLoS One. 2014;9:e87510. Medline:24489931 doi:10.1371/journal.pone.0087510

4 World Health Organization. The global elimination of congenital syphilis: rationale and strategy for action. Geneva: WHO; 2007.

5 UNAIDS. Global AIDS Monitoring 2018: Indicators for monitoring the 2016 United Nations Political Declaration on Ending AIDS. Geneva: UNAIDS; 2017.

6 World Health Organization. Global Health Observatory. Available: https://apps.who.int/gho/data/node.main.A1357STI?lang=en). Accessed: 18 February 2019.

7 World Health Organization. Global guidance on criteria and processes for validation: Elimination of Mother-to-Child Transmission of HIV and Syphilis. Geneva: WHO; 2017.

8 United Nations. Sustainable Development Goals. Available: https://sustainabledevelopment.un.org/?menu=1300. Accessed: 18 February 2019.

9 Victora C, Requejo J, Boerma T, Amouzou A, Bhutta ZA, Black RE, et al. Countdown to 2030 for reproductive, maternal, newborn, child, and adolescent health and nutrition. Lancet Glob Health. 2016;4:e775-6. Medline:27650656 doi:10.1016/S2214-109X(16)30204-2

10 World Health Organization. Global strategy for women's children's and adolescents' health. Available: https://www.who.int/life-course/publications/global-strategy-2016-2030/en/. Accessed: 18 March 2019.

11 UNDATA. Annual number of births (Births). Available: http://data.un.org/Data.aspx?d=SOWC&f=inID%3A75. Accessed 18 March 2019.

12 UNSTATS. UN Statistical Division, live births, deaths, and infant deaths, latest available year (2004-2018). Available: https://unstats.un.org/unsd/demographic-social/products/vitstats/seratab3.pdf. Accessed: 18 March 2019.

13 Blencowe H, Cousens S, Kamb M, Berman S, Lawn JE. Lives Saved Tool supplement detection and treatment of syphilis in pregnancy to reduce syphilis related stillbirths and neonatal mortality. BMC Public Health. 2011;11 Suppl 3:S9. Medline:21501460 doi:10.1186/1471-2458-11-S3-S9

14 Blencowe H, Cousens S, Jassir FB, Say L, Chou D, Mathers C, et al. Lancet Stillbirth Epidemiology Investigator Group. National, regional, and worldwide estimates of stillbirth rates in 2015, with trends from 2000: a systematic analysis. Lancet Glob Health. 2016;4:e98-108. Medline:26795602 doi:10.1016/S2214-109X(15)00275-2

15 World Health Organization. Sexual and Reproductive Health indicators database. Department of Reproductive Health and Research.

16 Gomez G, Newman LM, Mark J, Broutet N, Hawkes SJ. Untreated maternal syphilis and adverse outcomes of pregnancy: a systematic review and meta-analysis. Bull World Health Organ. 2013;91:217-26. Medline:23476094 doi:10.2471/BLT.12.107623

17 Ham DC, Newman L, Wijesooriya NS, Kamb M. Improving global estimates of syphilis in pregnancy by diagnostic test type: A systematic review and meta-analysis. Int J Gynaecol Obstet. 2015;130:S10-4. Medline:25963909 doi:10.1016/j.ijgo.2015.04.012

18 Nurse-Findlay S, Taylor MM, Savage M, Mello MB, Saliyou S, Lavayen M, et al. Supply, demand, and shortages of benzathine penicillin for treatment of syphilis: A market assessment. PLoS Med. 2017;14:e1002473. Medline:29281619 doi:10.1371/journal.pmed.1002473

19 World Health Organization. WHO recommendations on antenatal care of a positive pregnancy experience. Geneva: WHO; 2016.

20 World Health Organization. In vitro diagnostics and laboratory technology. Public reports of WHO prequalified IVDs. Available: https://www.who.int/diagnostics_laboratory/evaluations/pq-list/hiv_syphilis. Accessed: 18 March 2019.

21 Storey A, Seghers F, Pyne-Mercier L, Peeling RW, Owiredu MN, Taylor MM. Syphilis diagnosis and treatment during antenatal care: The potential catalytic impact of the dual HIV/Syphilis Rapid Diagnostic Test. Lancet Glob Health. 2019;7:e1006-8. Medline:31303285 doi:10.1016/S2214-109X(19)30248-7

22 Countdown to 2030. Countdown to 2030: Women's, Children's and Adolescent Health, homepage. Available: http://countdown2030.org/about/data. Assessed: 3 April 2019.

23 Baker U, Okuga M, Waiswa P, Manzi F, Peterson S, Hanson C. Bottlenecks in the implementation of essential screening tests in antenatal care: Syphilis, HIV, and anemia testing in rural Tanzania and Uganda. Int J Gynaecol Obstet. 2015;130:S43-50. Medline:26054252 doi:10.1016/j.ijgo.2015.04.017

24 Althabe F, Chomba E, Tshefu AK, Banda E, Belizán M, Bergel E, et al. A multifaceted intervention to improve syphilis screening and treatment in pregnant women in Kinshasa, Democratic Republic of the Congo and in Lusaka, Zambia: a cluster randomised controlled trial. Lancet Glob Health. 2019;7:e655-63. Medline:30910531 doi:10.1016/S2214-109X(19)30075-0

Basic maternal health care coverage among adolescents in 22 sub-Saharan African countries with high adolescent birth rate

Liliana Carvajal[1], Emily Wilson[2], Jennifer Harris Requejo[1], Holly Newby[3], Cristina de Carvalho Eriksson[4], Mengjia Liang[5], Mardieh Dennis[6], Fatima Gohar[7], Aline Simen-Kapeu[8], Priscilla Idele[9], Agbessi Amouzou[2]

[1] Data and Analytics Section, Division of Data, Analytics, Policy and Monitoring, United Nations Children's Fund UNICEF, HQ, New York, New York, USA

[2] Department of International Health, Johns Hopkins Bloomberg School of Public Health, Baltimore, Maryland, USA

[3] Independent consultant, Stockholm, Sweden.

[4] Health Section, Programme Division, UNICEF HQ, New York, New York, USA

[5] Population and Development Branch, Technical Division, United Nations Population Fund (UNFPA), New York, New York, USA

[6] London School of Hygiene and Tropical Medicine LSHTM, London, UK

[7] Regional Office for Eastern and Southern Africa ESARO, UNICEF , Nairobi, Kenya

[8] Regional Office for West and Central Africa, WCARO, UNICEF, Dakar, Senegal

[9] Office of Research-Innocenti, UNICEF Florence, Italy

Background In the sub-Saharan Africa region, the adolescent birth rate is the highest in the world, estimated at 100.5 births per 1000 women aged 15 to 19 years, and 2.4 times greater than the global average. This analysis examines coverage levels and gaps in basic maternal health care for adolescent mothers living in this region.

Methods We used data from national Demographic and Health Surveys (DHS) and Multiple Indicator Cluster Surveys (MICS) conducted between 2010 and 2016 in 22 of the sub-Saharan African Countdown to 2030 priority countries with adolescent birth rates above 100 in 2016. We analyzed 11 indicators of coverage of key services provided during the pre-pregnancy, pregnancy, delivery and postnatal period. We described the coverage level among adolescent girls aged 15-19 and women aged 20-49 for basic indicators in the continuum of care. We conducted a multilevel random effect logistic regression to quantify the association between the receipt of basic package of maternal care and woman's socio-demographic and socio-economic characteristics.

Results The median coverage of the basic package of maternal care among adolescents was extremely low, at 9.3%. Adolescent mothers who were in the highest household wealth quintile (odds ratio OR = 2.44, 95% confidence interval (CI) = 2.23-2.68), living in an urban area (OR = 1.25, 95% CI = 1.18-1.33) and having secondary education (OR = 1.61, 95% CI = 1.50-1.73) had greater odds of receiving the basic package of maternal health care as compared to those in the lowest wealth quintile, living in rural areas, and with no education respectively. Adolescent girls aged 15-17 and 18-19 had respectively 26% (OR = 0.74, 95% CI = 0.67-0.82) and 9% (OR = 0.91, 95% CI = 0.84-0.98) lower odds of receiving the basic package compared to women 20-49 years old. Child brides had 12% (OR = 0.88, 95% CI = 0.84-0.93) lower odds of receiving the basic package compared to women who were married after the age of 18.

Conclusion Coverage of basic maternal health care for adolescent mothers is inadequate in the countries with the highest adolescent birth rates in the world. Addressing the reproductive and maternal health needs of adolescents in sub-Saharan Africa is of critical importance, especially given projections that this region will experience the highest increases in adolescent births in the coming decades.

Globally, adolescents between the ages of 15 and 19 years comprise 8% of the population, or about 600 million [1]. Approximately 16 million girls aged 15 to 19 years and two million girls below 15 years of age give birth annually [2].

An estimated 11% of all global births are to adolescents aged 15 to 19 years [3]. Although the global adolescent birth rate decreased by 27% from 56.4 to 41.2 births per 1000 women aged 15-19 years between 2000 and 2020, progress was uneven and large disparities remain between world regions [4]. Adolescent births are concentrated in low and middle income countries, and particularly in sub-Saharan Africa, where over one in four adolescent girls gives birth before reaching 18 years [5]. Estimated at 100.5 births per 1000 women aged 15 to 19 years, the adolescent birth rate in sub-Saharan Africa is the highest in the world and 2.4 times greater than the global average [4].

Adolescent pregnancy and childbirth are linked to poor perinatal health outcomes and potential long-term negative economic and social consequences. Young adolescent mothers are at increased risk of death [3] and pregnancy-related morbidity, such as pre-eclampsia. The risk of adverse health outcomes is highest among young adolescents who give birth before the age of 15 years as compared to non-adolescent mothers [2,6,7]. Adolescent girls who become parents often faced pressure to discontinue their education, which reduces their employment prospects and puts them at greater risk of poverty [2,8,9]. Policies encouraging equal opportunities for educational attainment and for employment opportunities would likely help decrease the prevalence of adolescent pregnancy [10].

The negative social consequences of adolescent childbirth are often the same factors that place girls at increased risk of early and unintended pregnancy. Girls living in communities that are poorer, less educated, or rural are more likely to become adolescent mothers [11]. And these girls also experience greater challenges with accessing high quality maternal health services compared to their wealthier counterparts [12,13]. Adolescents face multiple barriers in accessing health care and information [14]. In many parts of the world, stigma associated with adolescent pregnancy, health services that are not responsive to adolescent needs, and low financial protection for adolescent mothers may contribute to insufficient coverage of essential maternal health services among this age group [15]. Although recent studies have shown that adolescent girls in low- and middle-income countries have a high unmet need for contraceptive services and often receive low-quality care, comparatively fewer studies have comprehensively examined the coverage, continuity, or quality of maternal care that adolescents receive once they become pregnant [16-19].

The World Health Organization(WHO) now recommends that all pregnant women receive a minimum of eight antenatal care (ANC) contacts, with the first contact occurring within the first three months of pregnancy; have a skilled attendant at birth; and receive routine postnatal health checks by a health provider within the first 48 hours of delivery [20,21]. Prior to 2016, WHO recommended that pregnant women receive a minimum of four visits [20]. Existing research on maternal health service use among adolescents in sub-Saharan Africa suggests that there is wide variation between countries; however, coverage tends to be insufficient and lower among adolescents than among older women. A study of antenatal care use in 13 West African countries found that only 62% of adolescent mothers aged 10-19 years received four or more antenatal visits for their first birth compared to 71% and 81% of women aged 20 to 24 years and 25 to 49 years, respectively [22]. Further, the study found that even among women who received at least four visits, adolescent mothers were less likely to have received recommended interventions for ANC such as blood pressure measurements, and urine and blood testing, and discussing potential pregnancy complications [22]. Similarly, an earlier study of 21 countries in sub-Saharan Africa found that adolescents aged 15-19 years were less likely to receive four or more antenatal visits, deliver in a health facility, and have a skilled birth attendant compared to women aged 20 years and older [23].

Given that sub-Saharan Africa is projected to experience the highest increase in the number of adolescent births between 2010 and 2030, it is imperative to better understand maternal health service use patterns among adolescents in this region and identify areas for programmatic action [11]. Low levels of coverage for maternal health services regardless of age highlight the need to dramatically improve outreach and service delivery overall in sub-Saharan Africa. Adolescents have unique needs which must be taken into account when designing and scaling up adolescent responsive programmes. The aim of this study is to describe coverage of key reproductive and maternal health indicators among adolescent mothers in 22 countries in sub-Saharan Africa with high adolescent birth rates and examine the influence of socioeconomic factors of receiving basic maternal health care.

METHODS

Data and study population

This study uses data from 22 countries in sub-Saharan Africa. These countries are 'Countdown to 2030' priority countries with high adolescent birth rates, defined as closest to 100 adolescent births per 1000 women aged 15 to 19 years in 2016, given that this is the highest regional average across SDG regions. Among the 25 countries meeting this criterion, 22 countries with a publicly available DHS or MICS conducted since 2010 were included in this analysis and all are in Sub-Saharan Africa (**Table 1**). Data used in these analyses included 18 Demographic and Health Surveys (DHS) and 4 Multiple Indicator Cluster Surveys (MICS) conducted in the period 2010-2016. The DHS and MICS are nationally representative, cross-sectional surveys using multi-stage cluster sampling. In each sampled household, individual questionnaires are administered to all women aged 15 to 49 years covering a range of topics including reproductive health, child health, nutrition, malaria, HIV/AIDS, etc. Both surveys use standardized questionnaires allowing for the analysis of outcomes across countries and surveys. In cases where more than one survey was conducted since 2010, the most recent survey was selected. The total sample comprised 22 135 adolescent girls aged 15-19 years in the households sampled across the 22 countries included in the analysis, with the largest sample in Nigeria (2053 adolescents) and the lowest in Zimbabwe (508 adolescents) (**Table 1**). We examined service coverage levels of all adolescent mothers who reported having at least one live birth in the two years preceding the survey.

Indicators and definitions

This study explored an initial set of 11 indicators related to intervention coverage and content of care for basic maternal health care: demand for family planning satisfied with modern methods, antenatal care contacts (first visit by 3rd trimester, at least four visits, and at least 8 visits); antenatal care content (receipt of all four selected interventions during ANC visits: blood pressure measured, having a blood sample taken, having a urine sample taken, and receiving tetanus toxoid), skilled birth attendant, institutional delivery, staying in health facility at least 24 hours after delivery, postnatal care visits for mother and baby and early initiation of breastfeeding. Descriptive results are presented in Table S1 of the **Online Supplementary Document**. The selection of these indicators was based on WHO recommendations for the antenatal, delivery and postnatal period [19,20,24].

Table 1. *Characteristics of countries and data sets used in analysis**

Country	Number of adolescents (15-19 age group) in the sample	Age specific fertility rate: 15-19 age group	Survey year	Survey type
Angola	1399	163	2015-2016	DHS
Burkina Faso	966	130	2010	DHS
Cameroon	566	128	2014	MICS
Central African Republic	595	229	2010	MICS
Chad	1472	179	2014-2015	DHS
Congo-Brazzaville	884	147	2011-2012	DHS
Côte d'Ivoire	581	129	2011-2012	DHS
Democratic Republic of Congo	1432	138	2013-2014	DHS
Gabon	595	114	2012	DHS
Guinea	649	146	2012	DHS
Guinea-Bissau	579	137	2014	MICS
Kenya	1311	96	2014	DHS
Liberia	720	149	2013	DHS
Malawi	1571	136	2015-2016	DHS
Mali	1333	178	2015	MICS
Mozambique	1081	167	2011	DHS
Niger	836	206	2012	DHS
Nigeria	2053	122	2013	DHS
Sierra Leone	1058	125	2013	DHS
Tanzania	841	132	2015-2016	DHS
Zambia	1105	141	2013-2014	DHS
Zimbabwe	508	110	2015	DHS
Total	22 135			

*Source: Survey data from Demographic and Health Surveys (DHS) and Multiple Indicators Cluster Surveys (MICS).

We defined the co-coverage of selected maternal and newborn health interventions that we referred to as basic package of maternal health care. Indicators included are related to service contact or interventions received during antenatal, delivery and postpartum period, based on WHO recommendations for care during these periods [21-23] and data availability. Thus, the basic package of maternal health care consists of the co-coverage of four indicators: having at least four antenatal care contacts, having received 4 key antenatal care content interventions (blood pressure measured, blood and urine sample taken, received tetanus toxoid injection), having had a skilled attendant at birth, and initiating breastfeeding within one hour of delivery. A woman received the basic maternal package when she received all four interventions or services contacts. Other indicators initially assessed in the descriptive part of the analysis were dropped from the basic package due to lack of data across all countries in the analysis. Although early initiation of breastfeeding is specific to newborns, we used it as a proxy for maternal intrapartum care given the measurement issues and data availability for these indicators. A total of 3 399 had missing data to accurately calculate the basic package indicator and full set of demographic characteristics, and so were dropped in the demographic tables.

We considered socio-demographic factors with known association with the coverage indicators above. These include age of woman at time of delivery, household wealth, area of residence (urban or rural), education, parity, and child marriage. We defined child marriage using women's age at first marriage or union. Women who were currently married or in union and less than 18 years of age, as well as women who were 18 or older whose age at first marriage or union was less than 18, were classified as child brides.

Statistical analysis

We described the level of the coverage indicators, disaggregated by age groups, considering adolescents aged 15-19 years old and older women aged 20-49. Point estimates and 95% confidence intervals were computed. We ran a multilevel logistic regression model with random effects fitted for country in pooled data set, to explore the association between the receipt of the basic package of maternal health care and age group, controlling for socio-demographic factors. We exponentiated the coefficients and confidence intervals to get odds ratios for each fixed effects covariate, and examined between country variance from the random effects results.

All results were weighted and adjusted to account for survey multi-stage sampling design. We conducted all analyses in R version 3.3.1 (Foundation for Statistical Computing, Vienna, Austria).

RESULTS

Descriptive analysis

Characteristics of the study population

Across the 22 countries included in the analysis, 22 135 adolescents had a live birth in the two years preceding the survey. Out of this total 1806 (9.3%) received the basic package of maternal health care. Among the adolescents in the analysis 46% were among the poorest two quintiles and 32% were among the richest two quintiles. In terms of residence, 69% live in urban areas and 31% in rural areas. In terms of education achievement, 28% had no education, 40% started primary education and 30% started secondary education (**Table 2**).

Table 2. *Demographic table by age of woman at time of delivery and receiving basic maternal health care package**

Covariates	Age group 15-19						Age group 20-49					
	Received basic package						Received basic package					
	Yes		No		Total		Yes		No		Total	
	N	%	N	%	N	%	N	%	N	%	N	%
Household wealth:												
Poorest	275	15.2	4059	24.0	4334	23.1	960	12.7	15 167	22.6	16 127	21.6
Poorer	329	18.2	3947	23.3	4276	22.8	1076	14.3	14 712	21.9	15 788	21.1
Middle	409	22.6	3761	22.2	4170	22.3	1369	18.2	13 869	20.7	15 238	20.4
Richer	432	23.9	3109	18.4	3541	18.9	1824	24.2	12 706	18.9	14 530	19.5
Richest	361	20.0	2054	12.1	2415	12.9	2305	30.6	10 705	15.9	13 010	17.4
Area of residence:												
Urban	1008	55.8	11 963	70.7	12 971	69.2	3661	48.6	46 114	68.7	49 775	66.6
Rural	798	44.2	4967	29.3	5765	30.8	3873	51.4	21 045	31.3	24 918	33.4
Highest level of education:												
No education	333	18.4	4998	29.5	5331	28.5	2118	28.1	28 102	41.9	30 220	40.5
Started primary education	680	37.7	6950	41.1	7630	40.7	2257	30.0	23 068	34.4	25 325	33.9
Started secondary education/higher	793	43.9	4981	29.4	5774	30.8	3156	41.9	15 978	23.8	19 134	25.6
First time mother:												
No	497	27.5	5584	33.0	6081	32.5	6307	83.7	61 108	91.0	67 415	90.3
Yes	1309	72.5	11 346	67.0	12 655	67.5	1227	16.3	6051	9.0	7278	9.7
Child marriage:												
No	863	47.8	6370	37.6	7233	38.6	4869	64.6	35 891	53.4	40 760	54.6
Yes	943	52.2	10 560	62.4	11 503	61.4	2665	35.4	31 268	46.6	33 933	45.4
Total	1806		16 930		18 736	100.0	7534		67 159		74 693	100.0

*The number of adolescents in the whole study is 22 135. Of those, 3399 are missing data to accurately calculate the basic package indicator, and so were dropped in the demographic tables. Source: authors' analysis using data from DHS and MICS surveys included in the analysis.

*The number of adolescents in the whole study is 22 135. Of those, 3399 are missing data to accurately calculate the basic package indicator, and so were dropped in the demographic tables. Source: authors' analysis using data from DHS and MICS surveys included in the analysis.

Service use and practices across the maternal health continuum

Coverage of basic maternal health care indicators

Among adolescent mothers, the median coverage for at least 4 ANC visits was estimated at 50.6% (95% CI = 47.1%-54.2%), 40.9% (95% CI = 36.5%-45.4%) for specific routine services (blood test, blood pressure measurement, urine testing and neonatal tetanus vaccination), 65% (95% CI = 61.5%-68.9%) had a skilled attendant assisting the delivery of their last child and 45.7% (95% CI = 41.3%-50.2%) initiated breastfeeding within the first hour after delivery. However, only 9.3% (95% CI = 6.7%-11.7%) of them received the full set of all these interventions or services which defines the basic package of maternal health care (Table S1 in the **Online Supplementary Document**).

Coverage of the other maternal health indicators not in the package was also low. The median percentage of adolescents aged 15-19 who reported having demand for family planning satisfied was 25.6% (95% CI = 20.6%-30.8%). The median percentage of adolescents who started ANC during their first trimester of pregnancy was only 24.9% (95% CI = 20.3%-29.5%) and only 3.5% (95% CI = 1.9%- 4.9%) had eight or more antenatal care contacts.

There was substantial cross-country variation across indicators included in this analysis. Country specific coverage of additional maternal health indicators are included in Table S1 in the **Online Supplementary Document.**

Figure 1 displays boxplots of the proportion of women who received each intervention included in the basic package, stratified in three 3 age groups: adolescents 15-17, 18-19 and older women 20-49. The dots represent country-level proportions, while the boxplots show the median, interquartile range, mini-

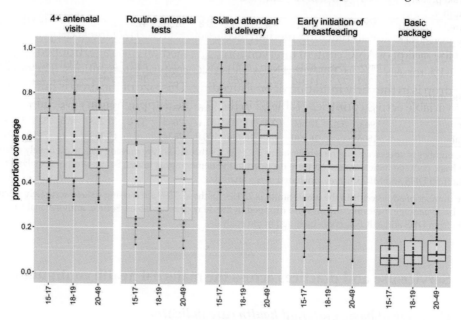

Figure 1. *Coverage of basic maternal health care package across all 22 countries for all age groups younger adolescents (15-17 years), older adolescent (18-19 years) and older women (20-49 years). Figure presents the interquartile ranges of the coverage of the basic package of essential maternal care among 3 age groups: 15-17, 15-19 and 20-49. The dots represent country-level estimates, while the box plots represent the median, interquartile range, and minimum and maximum values across countries. The basic package is composed of 4 main interventions: 4+ antenatal care visits; ANC care (receipt of routine tests such as urine and blood test, blood pressure measured, tetanus toxoid injection); skilled attendant at time of delivery; and early initiation of breastfeeding. The denominator for the components of the basic package in this figure is women with live birth in last 2 years (n = 22 135 adolescents). Source: authors' analysis using data from DHS and MICS surveys included in the analysis.*

mum and maximum values across countries. Median coverage of indicators included in the basic package is low across the board. Younger adolescents have the lowest median coverage value of three out of the four components of the basic package except for skilled birth attendant. The co-coverage of the four indicators included in the basic package is extremely low and similar across the three age groups.

In order to understand the source of the low coverage values among adolescents that we observed for the basic package, we visualized the component indicators in a cascade with each step adding one indicator at a time, starting from ANC4 (**Figure 2**). The cascade assumes a continuum of care from ANC4 to early initiation of breastfeeding (EIBF) although the receipt of the ANC content interventions may not necessarily require four ANC contacts. However, the cascade shows where adolescents are more likely to drop off on the continuum between ANC and EIBF. Starting with the ANC4 as it is the component that had highest coverage, across countries, the coverage drops as each of the components is added reaching median levels below 10%. The largest drop was in the receipt of ANC content interventions. The median coverage dropped from 61% for ANC4+ to 28% for ANC4 and ANC content interventions. The next drop is in the early initiation of breastfeeding. This size of the drop is however variable across countries (Table S2 in the **Online Supplementary Document**).

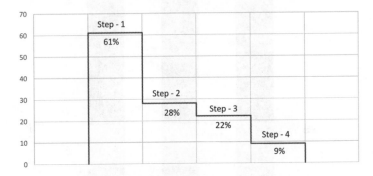

Figure 2. *Cascade of loss of coverage (median across countries) from ANC4 to early initiation of breastfeeding among adolescent mothers 15-19. The basic package is composed of 4 interventions, which are differentially limiting among adolescents by country. Each dot represents the coverage in each of the countries in the analysis. Step 1 shows the proportion who received 4+ antenatal visits; Step 2 shows the proportion of adolescents who received both 4+ antenatal visits and routine antenatal tests (urine test, blood test, blood pressure measurement, and tetanus toxoid injection); Step 3 shows the proportion who received 4+ antenatal visits, routine tests, and had a skilled attendant at delivery; Step 4 shows the proportion who received 4+ antenatal visits, routine tests, had a skilled attendant at delivery, and initiated breastfeeding within the first hour after birth. Source: authors' analysis using data from DHS and MICS surveys included in the analysis.*

For a country like Congo the drop went from 77% ANC4+ to 46% when ANC content is added. Coverage remained mostly unchanged when skilled birth at delivery was included successively. Additional drop was observed when early initiation of breastfeeding was included. This pattern was observed in many countries in the analysis.

Figure 3 presents the co-coverage of the four indicators included in the basic package of maternal health care by the number of interventions or services that women across three age groups received. For 1, 2, 3 interventions or services, it refers to any combination of the 4 included in the basic package. The percentage distribution of each count is presented by age of the mother at time of delivery (15-17, 18-19 and 20-49). On average, less than 10% of women across the three age groups received zero maternal health interventions or services and 21% received at least one. Between 32 and 34 percent of women received any two interventions or services and between 28 and 29% received any three. About 36% of younger adolescents compared to 39% of older adolescents and adult women received three or more interventions or service contacts. However, only 9 to 10% of women across all age groups received all four basic maternal health interventions or services.

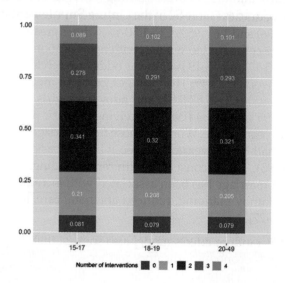

Figure 3. *Co-coverage of basic maternal health care interventions and services. Distribution of number of interventions among women whose basic package components can be evaluated N = 18 736. Interventions include any combination of the following interventions: receiving 4+ antenatal visits; receiving routine antenatal tests (urine test, blood test, blood pressure measurement, and tetanus toxoid injection); having had a skilled attendant at delivery; having initiated breastfeeding within the first hour after birth. Source: authors' analysis using data from DHS and MICS surveys included in the analysis.*

Factors associated with receiving the basic maternal health package

To better understand the reasons for poor continuity of maternal care, we examined available social and economic factors which could potentially be associated with receiving the basic maternal health care package, namely age of woman at time of delivery, household wealth, area of residence, education, parity, and child marriage. Higher household wealth, urban residence, and higher educational achievement, were positively associated with receiving the basic maternal health package. On the other hand, younger age and having been a child bride were negatively associated with receiving the basic maternal health package. To be included in the inferential analysis, individuals had to have data for each of the components of the basic maternal health package outcome as well as each covariate, reducing the sample for the subsequent pooled analysis across all age groups to 18 736 women whose most recent birth was when they were ages 15-19 and 74 693 women 20-49.

As presented in **Table 3** and **Figure 4**, women in the highest household wealth quintile had 2.44 times higher odds (95% CI = 2.23-2.68) of receiving the basic maternal care package compared to women in the lowest household wealth quintile. Living in an urban area was associated with 1.25 times greater odds (95% CI = 1.18-1.33) of receiving the basic maternal health care package and starting primary education and secondary education were associated with 1.28 (95% CI = 1.20-1.36) and 1.61 (95% CI = 1.50-1.73) times greater odds of receiving the basic package compared to women with no education. In contrast, adolescent girls aged 15-17 and 18-19 had lower odds of receiving the basic package as compared to women 20-49. The younger group of mothers had 26% lower odds (OR = 0.74, 95% CI = 0.67-0.82) and adolescent girls 18-19 had 9% lower odds (OR = 0.91, 95% CI = 0.84-0.98) of receiving the basic package as compared to women 20-49 years of age. Women whose first marriage occurred before the age of 18 years had 12% lower odds of receiving the basic package (OR = 0.88, 95% CI = 0.84-0.93). This is consistent with recent findings in the literature in which girl child marriage has been associated with increased fertility and reduced modern family planning, reduced antenatal care, and lower levels of safe delivery [25-27].

Results from our random effects model also suggest that the relationship between various socioeconomic indicators and access to the basic package of maternal care varies by country. The variance for the random effect of country tells us how much of the covariate variance is explained by differences between countries. The among-country variance, 0.56, is larger than the magnitude of all of the treatment effects, except for the intercept (-3.04) and the fourth and fifth wealth quintiles (0.60, and 0.89, respectively), and this may reflect differences between countries in the norms, policies, and legislation pertaining to adolescent pregnancy and adolescents' access to sexual and reproductive health services responsive to their needs.

Table 3. *Determinants of receiving the basic maternal health care package**

	Adjusted†	
	aOR† (95% CI)	P-value
Age (years) of woman at time of delivery:		
15-17	0.74 (0.67, 0.82)	<0.001
18-19	0.91 (0.84, 0.98)	<0.001
20-49	reference	
Wealth quintile:		
Poorest	reference	
Poorer	1.12 (1.03, 1.21)	<0.001
Middle	1.38 (1.28, 1.50)	<0.001
Richer	1.82 (1.68, 1.98)	<0.001
Richest	2.44 (2.23, 2.68)	<0.001
Area of residence:		
Rural	reference	
Urban	1.25 (1.18, 1.33)	<0.001
Highest level of education:		
No education	reference	
Started primary education	1.28 (1.20, 1.36)	<0.001
Started secondary education/higher	1.61 (1.50, 1.73)	<0.001
First time mother:		
No	reference	
Yes	1.31 (1.23, 1.40)	<0.001
Child marriage:		
No	reference	
Yes	0.88 (0.84, 0.93)	<0.001

aOR – adjusted odds ratio, CI – confidence interval
*We fit a logistic regression model with fixed effects of age, wealth, residence, education, parity, and child marriage, and random effects for countries. Odds ratios for fixed effects are shown here. Women who did not have data for all covariates were excluded from this analysis. Odds overlapping with 1 do not differ statistically from the reference group, while ranges that fall below one decrease the odds of getting the basic package, and covariates with ranges higher than one increase the odds of getting the basic package. Source: authors' analysis using data from DHS and MICS surveys included in the analysis. Odds ratios (OR): unadjusted associations between the variable and the outcome.
†Adjusted odds ratio (aOR): odds ratio adjusted for all other variables reported in the table.

DISCUSSION

We examined coverage of key reproductive and maternal health services and determinants of receiving a basic package of maternal care among adolescents and older women in 22 sub-Saharan African countries with the highest adolescent birth rates in the world. Overall, the findings showed that even basic, yet critical services along and across the maternal health continuum, are not all reaching most women and particularly adolescents: Across these countries, the co-coverage of the four indicators included in the basic package of maternal services was only 9.3% (95% CI = 6.7%-11.7%) of adolescents who delivered in the two years preceding the surveys This co-coverage proportion ranges from 2% (95% CI = 1%-3.1%) of adolescents in Mali to 31.7% (95% CI = 26.7%-36.7%) in Liberia. Although coverage of many maternal health services has improved

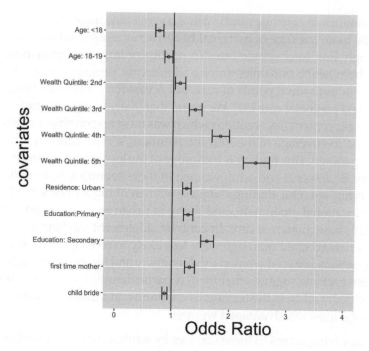

Figure 4. *Odds ratios of the determinants of receiving the basic e package. Adjusted odds ratio (aOR): odds ratio adjusted for all other variables reported in the table. Reference categories: For age of woman at time of delivery: age 20-49; for wealth quintiles: 1ˢᵗ quintile; for area of residence: is rural; for education: no education; for first time mother: not being a first time mother; and for child marriage: not having experience child marriage. Source: authors' analysis using data from DHS and MICS surveys included in the analysis.*

over the past two decades, progress towards increasing access to adolescent responsive maternal health services must also be accelerated in order to meet SDG aims of achieving universal coverage of maternal care for all women, including adolescent mothers. This is particularly important given the projected increase in adolescent births over the coming decade. An estimated 12.8 million adolescent girls have an unmet need for family planning in low- and middle-income countries, and this is projected to increase to 15 million by 2030 [28]. As part of efforts to reduce adolescent birth rates and improve maternal outcomes, improving knowledge of, access to and use of family planning services are essential. Available data on levels and trends of family planning indicators, including demand for family planning satisfied, contraceptive use and met need for spacing, indicate that adolescents do not have enough access to modern contraceptive methods [29-31]. These findings are consistent with the results in this analysis which show insufficient coverage of demand for family planning satisfied with modern methods: median of 25.6% (95C%CI: 20.6%-30.8%) among adolescents 15-19 years of age.

Our continuum of care approach with a co-coverage measure of four indicators in the basic package of maternal health services allowed us to uncover a surprisingly low co-coverage rate. To maximize improvements in maternal and newborn health outcomes among adolescents, progress must not only be measured at individual points of care, but across the continuum of antenatal, delivery and postnatal care [32]. We found that many women are not receiving all ANC basic content interventions which was most responsible for most of the drop in the co-coverage of the four interventions/service contract included in the basic package. This finding is indicative of the low quality of antenatal care receive by adolescents and adult women in these countries, where adolescent fertility is highest. Our findings suggest women of higher household wealth, higher educational attainment, and living in urban areas were more likely to receive this basic maternal care. In contrast, adolescent mothers and the ones who experienced child marriage were less likely to receive the basic package. The associations between women's vulnerability and lower use of the basic maternal care package suggests that there is particular need to better understand and specifically address the barriers to continuity and quality of maternal care faced by the most disadvantaged women.

While improving access to these services by adolescents is essential, a critical strategy remains in addressing the prevalence of child marriage practices that lead to premature childbearing. Other strategies to be considered for reducing adolescent birth rate include addressing discriminatory gender and social norms as well as economic inequality, so that adolescent girls have the same opportunities as boys to be educated and to reach their full potential [33].

An essential component to increasing the chances that women receive all of the recommended maternal health services during pregnancy is ensuring that they make the minimum recommended number of ANC contacts [34]. For a positive pregnancy experience, WHO recommends that many of the interventions be initiated during the first trimester of pregnancy. Therefore, it is critical to develop strategies to facilitate earlier ANC initiation among pregnant adolescents [20].

Given that the majority of maternal deaths are preventable with routine, life-saving interventions and an estimated one third of maternal deaths are due to complications that arise during labor, childbirth, and the immediate post-partum period, the large proportions of adolescent mothers delivering under sub-optimal conditions is contributing to poor maternal outcomes in countries with high adolescent birth rates [24]. Efforts to accelerate progress towards improved maternal health by 2030 must therefore focus both on improving appropriate service-seeking behaviors, as well as ensuring that all adolescents receive high quality, respectful care responding to their needs when they seek maternity care.

As immediate breastfeeding initiation is associated with improved newborn survival, long-term breastfeeding practices, child outcomes, health outcomes for the mother, and interventions to improve quality of maternal care, must include training on breastfeeding counseling [35].

Information on country adoption of legislation permitting adolescents to access contraceptive services without parental or spousal consent also shows that many countries with high adolescent fertility are also those with low adoption of such legislation. For instance, out of the 22 countries in the analysis, only eight countries have a policy in place for contraceptive services for adolescents without spousal or parental consent [31]. Similarly, many countries with high adolescent birth rates tend to have weak enforcement of or no introduction of legislation on the minimum age of marriage [31]. Also, gender and social norms play a key role in the tendency towards child marriage and early childbearing. For instance, these practices vary across countries in the Sahel region and countries in the coastal areas of West Africa. Additional research is therefore necessary to better understand the context-specific barriers to women's access to essential and quality maternal care, and to develop effective interventions relevant for different contexts and the difference in patterns brought by country or region-specific social and gender norms.

This study has some limitations. As this is a secondary analysis of DHS and MICS data, data availability played an important role in shaping the study design. This affected both the countries and indicators included in the analysis. For instance, although interventions such as HIV testing, iron supplementation, breastfeeding counseling, deworming, and intermittent preventive treatment of malaria are all important components of antenatal care, we were unable to include them in our analyses due to lack of availability of data for these indicators across all of the study countries. Given the measurement issues and data availability of the postnatal care indicators, early initiation of breastfeeding was used as a proxy of postnatal care in the basic package of maternal health services. Additionally, all of the outcomes in the study rely on self-reported survey data, which may be subject to recall bias specifically in regard to women's ability to correctly recall specific check-ups during the antenatal period or intrapartum period. Despite these limitations, this study is the first one analyzing a basic package of services using nationally representative data sets in 22 countries with a sample size of over 18 000 adolescents in sub-Saharan African countries with high childbearing among adolescents. The conclusions therefore are generalizable to other countries with similar characteristics. Our study provides useful insights into maternal health service use and content of care among adolescent girls and women in countries with high adolescent birth rates.

CONCLUSIONS

Our findings demonstrate that the coverage of basic maternal health services for adolescent mothers 15-19 is insufficient in the countries with the highest adolescent birth rates in the world. Drivers of poor maternal health outcomes are multi-faceted and may vary across and within countries. Addressing the specific needs of adolescents, however, is of critical importance, especially in sub-Saharan Africa where adolescent births are expected to increase in the coming decades. Reducing the burden of maternal mortality will therefore require an integrated, comprehensive approach to ensure that reproductive and adolescent responsive health services are made available, accessible, and acceptable to adolescent girls and young women in need at all points through-out the reproductive, maternal, and child health continuum.

Acknowledgements: The authors acknowledge the support from the Countdown to 2030 coverage working group members in terms of facilitating discussions and presentation of preliminary results at technical meetings. The authors would also like to thank Claudia Cappa and Colleen Murray Gaston from UNICEF HQ (Data and Analytics Section/ DAPM) for their advice related to child marriage data.

Disclaimer: The findings and conclusions in this report are those of the authors and do not necessarily represent the official position of the respective organization.

Funding: This work was funded by the Bill & Melinda Gates Foundation through separate grants to the Countdown to 2030 and the Data and Analytics Section of UNICEF-New York.

Authorship contributions: LCA and AA conceived and designed the analysis plan and led the analysis. LCA composed the initial draft. EW carried out the analysis and helped shape all the analytical components. MD drafted parts of the paper including literature review. AA and JHR provided analytical guidance. LCA, EW, JHR, HN, CCE ML, FG, ASK PI and AA reviewed drafts and provided inputs. All authors approved the final draft.

Competing interests: The authors have completed the ICMJE Unified Competing Interest form (available upon request from the corresponding author) and declare no conflict of interest.

Additional material
Online Supplementary Document

Reference
1 United Nations Department of Economic and Social Affairs Population Division. World Population Prospects: The 2019 Revision. vol. Volume I. 2019. POP/DB/WPP/ Rev.2019/INT/F03-1.
2 United Nations Population Fund (UNFPA). Girlhood, not motherhood preventing adolescent pregnancy. New York: UNFPA; 2015.
3 World Health Organization. Global Accelerated Action for the Health of Adolescents (AA-HA!) Guidance to Support Country Implementation. Geneva: WHO; 2017.

4   United Nations Economic and Social Council. Progress towards the Sustainable Development Goals: Report of the Secretary-General, Supplementary Information. 2020. E/2020/57.

5   United Nations Children's Fund (UNICEF). The state of the world's children 2019: Children, food and nutrition. Growing well in a changing world. New York: UNICEF. 2019.

6   Neal S, Mahendra S, Bose K, et al. The causes of maternal mortality in adolescents in low and middle income countries: a systematic review of the literature. BMC Pregnancy Childbirth. 2016;16:352. Medline:27836005 doi:10.1186/s12884-016-1120-8

7   Ganchimeg T, Ota E, Morisaki N, et al. Pregnancy and childbirth outcomes among adolescent mothers: a World Health Organization multicountry study. BJOG. 2014;121 Suppl 1:40-8. Medline:24641534 doi:10.1111/1471-0528.12630

8   Pradhan R, Wynter K, Fisher J. Factors associated with pregnancy among adolescents in low-income and lower middle-income countries: a systematic review. J Epidemiol Community Health. 2015;69:918-24. Medline:26034047 doi:10.1136/jech-2014-205128

9   Patton GC, Sawyer SM, Santelli JS, et al. Our future: a Lancet commission on adolescent health and wellbeing. Lancet. 2016;387:2423-78. Medline:27174304 doi:10.1016/S0140-6736(16)00579-1

10 United Nations Children's Fund (UNICEF). Health Equity Report 2016: Analysis of reproductive, maternal, newborn, child and adolescent health inequities in Latin America and the Caribbean to inform policymaking. New York: UNICEF; 2016.

11 United Nations Population Fund (UNFPA). Adolescent Pregnancy: A Review of the Evidence. New York: UNFPA; 2013.

12 Graham W, Woodd S, Byass P, et al. Diversity and divergence: the dynamic burden of poor maternal health. Lancet. 2016;388:2164-75. Medline:27642022 doi:10.1016/S0140-6736(16)31533-1

13 Campbell OMR, Calvert C, Testa A, et al. The scale, scope, coverage, and capability of childbirth care. Lancet. 2016;388:2193-208. Medline:27642023 doi:10.1016/S0140-6736(16)31528-8

14 Plan International. UNICEF, WHO and others. 2019 Adolescent Health: The Missing Population in Universal Health Coverage 2019. Available: https://plan-uk.org/blogs/adolescents-the-missing-population-in-universal-health-coverage. Accessed: 1 June 2019.

15 Tylee A, Haller DM, Graham T, et al. Youth-friendly primary-care services: how are we doing and what more needs to be done? Lancet. 2007;369:1565-73. Medline:17482988 doi:10.1016/S0140-6736(07)60371-7

16 Woog V, Singh S, Browne A, et al. Adolescent Women's Need for and Use of Sexual and Reproductive Health Services in Developing Countries. New York: 2015.

17 Dennis ML, Radovich E, Wong KLM, et al. Pathways to increased coverage: an analysis of time trends in contraceptive need and use among adolescents and young women in Kenya, Rwanda, Tanzania, and Uganda. Reprod Health. 2017;14:130. Medline:29041936 doi:10.1186/s12978-017-0393-3

18 Radovich E, Dennis ML, Wong KLM, et al. Who Meets the Contraceptive Needs of Young Women in Sub-Saharan Africa? J Adolesc Heal. 2017:1–8.

19 Darroch JE, Woog V, Bankole A, et al. Adding it up: Costs and benefits of meeting the contraceptive needs of adolescents. Guttmacher Institute. 2016 May. 2016:1–16.

20 World Health Organization. WHO Recommendation on antenatal care for positive pregnancy experience. Geneva: WHO; 2016.

21 World Health Organization. WHO recommendations on postnatal care of the mother and newborn 2013. Geneva: WHO; 2013.

22 Owolabi OO, Wong KLM, Dennis ML, et al. Comparing the use and content of ante-natal care in adolescent and older first-time mothers in 13 countries of west Africa: a cross-sectional analysis of Demographic and Health Surveys. Lancet Child Adolesc Health. 2017;1:203-12. Medline:30169169 doi:10.1016/S2352-4642(17)30025-1

23 Magadi MA, Agwanda AO, Obare FO. A comparative analysis of the use of maternal health services between teenagers and older mothers in sub-Saharan Africa: evidence from Demographic and Health Surveys (DHS). Soc Sci Med. 2007;64:1311-25. Medline:17174017 doi:10.1016/j.socscimed.2006.11.004

24 World Health Organization. Intrapartum care for a positive childbirth experience. Geneva: WHO; 2018.

25 Godha D, Hotchkiss D, Gage AJ, et al. Association Between Child Marriage and Reproductive Health Outcomes and Service Utilization: A Multi-Country Study From South Asia. J Adolesc Health. 2013;52:552-8. Medline:23608719 doi:10.1016/j.jadohealth.2013.01.021

26 Nasrullah M, Muazzam S, Bhutta ZA, et al. Girl Child Marriage and Its Effect on Fertility in Pakistan: Findings from Pakistan Demographic and Health Survey, 2006-2007. Matern Child Health J. 2014;18:534-43. Medline:23580067 doi:10.1007/s10995-013-1269-y

27 Raj A, Saggurti N, Balaiah D, et al. Prevalence of child marriage and its eff ect on fertility and fertility-control outcomes of young women in India: a cross-sectional, observational study. Lancet. 2009;373:1883-9. Medline:19278721 doi:10.1016/S0140-6736(09)60246-4

28 United Nations Population Fund (UNFPA). Universal Access to Reproductive Health: Progress and Challenges 2016. New York: UNFPA; 2016.

29 Kalamar AM, Tunçalp Ö, Hindin MJ. Developing strategies to address contraceptive needs of adolescents: exploring patterns of use among sexually active adolescents in 46 low- and middle-income countries. Contraception. 2018;98:36-40. Medline:29550455 doi:10.1016/j.contraception.2018.03.016

30 United Nations Department of Economic and Social Affairs Statistics Division. Indicator 3.7.1: Proportion of women of reproductive age (aged 15-49 years) who have their need for family planning satisfied with modern methods. Available: https://unstats.un.org/sdgs/metadata/files/Metadata-03-07-01.pdf. Accessed: 13 August 2019.

31 United Nations Children's Fund, World Health Organization. Tracking progress towards universal coverage for women's, children's and adolescents' health. Countdown to 2030: Maternal, Newborn and Child Survival: The 2017 Report. 2017. New York: UNICEF; 2017.

32 Kerber KJ, de Graft-Johnson JE, Bhutta ZA, et al. Continuum of care for maternal, newborn, and child health: from slogan to service delivery. Lancet. 2007;370:1358-69. Medline:17933651 doi:10.1016/S0140-6736(07)61578-5

33 United Nations Children's Fund (UNICEF). Adolescent girls' health and well-being in West and Central Africa. Available at: https://data.unicef.org/resources/adolescent-girls-health-and-well-being-in-west-and-central-africa/. Accessed: 13 August 2019.

34 Benova L, Tunçalp Ö, Moran AC, et al. Not just a number: examining coverage and content of antenatal care in low-income and middle-income countries. BMJ Glob Health. 2018;3:e000779. Medline:29662698 doi:10.1136/bmjgh-2018-000779

35 UNICEF, World Health Organization. Capture the moment - early initiation of breast-feeding: the best start for every newborn. New York: UNICEF; 2018.

Examining coverage, content, and impact of maternal nutrition interventions: the case for quality-adjusted coverage measurement

Naima T Joseph[1], Ellen Piwoz[2], Dennis Lee[3], Address Malata[4], Hannah H Leslie[5]; on behalf of the Countdown Coverage Technical Working Group

[1] Division of Maternal Fetal Medicine, Department of Gynecology and Obstetrics, Emory University School of Medicine, Atlanta, Georgia, USA

[2] Bill and Melinda Gates Foundation, Seattle, Washington, USA

[3] Department of Health Policy and Management, Harvard TH Chan School of Public Health, Boston, Massachusetts, USA

[4] Malawi University of Science and Technology, Limbe, Malawi

[5] Department of Global Health and Population, Harvard TH Chan School of Public Health, Boston, Massachusetts, USA

Background Reductions in neonatal mortality remain stagnant, despite gains in health care access and utilization. Nutrition interventions during antenatal care (ANC) and in the immediate postpartum period are associated with improved neonatal outcomes. Adjusting coverage estimates for the quality of care provided yields greater insight into health system performance and potential population health benefits of accessing care. In this cross-sectional study, we adjust maternity care coverage measures for quality of nutrition interventions to determine the impact on infant birth weight and breastfeeding.

Methods We used household data from the Malawi 2013-2014 Multiple Indicator Cluster Survey to assess use of maternal health services and direct observations of ANC and delivery from the 2013 Service Provision Assessment to measure nutrition interventions provided. We adjusted coverage measures combining self-reported utilization of care with the likelihood of receipt of nutrition interventions. Using adjusted log-linear regression, we estimated the associations of these nutrition quality-adjusted metrics with infant birthweight and immediate breastfeeding.

Results Health facility data provided over 2500 directly observed clinical encounters and household data provided 7385 individual reports of health care utilization and outcomes. Utilization of ANC and facility-delivery was high. Women received nutrition-related interventions considerably less often than they sought care: over the course of ANC women received a median of 1.6 interventions on iron, 1 instance of nutrition counseling, and 0.06 instances of breastfeeding counseling. Nutrition quality-adjusted ANC coverage was associated with a reduced risk of low birthweight (adjusted relative risk [ARR] 0.87, 95% confidence interval (CI) = 0.79, 0.96) and increased likelihood of immediate breastfeeding (ARR = 1.04, 95% CI = 1.02, 1.07); nutrition quality-adjusted post-delivery care was also associated with greater uptake of immediate breastfeeding (ARR = 1.08, 95% CI = 1.02, 1.14). Based on these models, delivering nutrition interventions consistently within the existing level of coverage would decrease population prevalence of low birthweight from 13.7% to 10.8% and increase population prevalence of immediate breastfeeding from 75.9% to 86.0%.

Conclusions Linking household survey data to health service provision assessments demonstrates that despite high utilization of maternal health services in Malawi, low provision of nutrition interventions is undermining infant health. Substantial gains in newborn health are possible in Malawi if quality of existing services is strengthened.

Despite the dramatic declines in overall child mortality in low- and middle-income countries, progress towards reduction in neonatal mortality remains slow. With an estimated 2.7 million annual deaths, neonatal mortality now comprises 60% of deaths in the first year of life and 40% of deaths in children under 5 [1,2].

Maternal and childhood undernutrition is thought to underlie 45% of neonatal mortality [3-5]. Interventions to improve maternal and infant nutrition such as dietary counseling, iron supplementation, and immediate/exclusive breastfeeding, have been associated with improved pregnancy and neonatal outcomes [1,6-10]. It is estimated that these interventions could avert more than 800 000 deaths in children under age 5 each year [11]. Iron supplementation has been demonstrated to reduce low birth weight, and immediate breastfeeding is associated with reduced neonatal mortality [1,12]. In addition to neonatal outcomes, breastfeeding has been associated with multiple child health benefits, including reduced overall child mortality, as well as reduction in childhood obesity, asthma, diabetes, and infection [13,14]. Maternal benefits include reductions in type II diabetes and in breast and ovarian cancer [13]. Failure to counsel women on the proximal and long-lasting maternal, neonatal, and child health benefits of iron supplementation and breastfeeding during antenatal care represents missed opportunity for improving long-term maternal and child health. Yet, antenatal coverage and counseling to support these practices are not consistently delivered or measured [1,12].

In 2016, the World Health Organization (WHO) reviewed their antenatal care (ANC) guidelines and reaffirmed their recommendations for dietary counseling, maternal iron supplementation, and exclusive breastfeeding within the context of routine ANC [15]. Additionally, WHO updated their guidelines to increase the frequency of ANC contacts from four to eight, emphasizing the importance of ANC in improving neonatal health outcomes [15]. Utilization of ANC services is associated with reduced probability of adverse neonatal outcomes such as mortality, low birth weight, and stunting [16]. The prioritization of increased access to health facilities and health care coverage during the Millennium Development Goal era led to dramatic increase in ANC utilization [17,18]. By 2015, 90% of women in the countries with 95% of global maternal and child mortality attended at least one ANC visit [17]; over half of women attended at least 4 ANC visits, and 3 out of 4 women delivered with a skilled birth attendant [19]. However, decreases in neonatal mortality did not keep pace with increased utilization of care; annual declines in neonatal mortality will need to double in high-mortality countries to achieve ambitious global targets by 2030 [19].

Analyses of the Demographic and Health Surveys (DHS) and self-reported evaluation on ANC content revealed missed opportunities to improve nutrition and breastfeeding in pregnant women. The focus on improving access to ANC, without ensuring adequate content of care, is insufficient to reducing adverse neonatal outcomes [9,20-24]. A recent analysis of health care-amenable mortality estimated that the majority (657 555 of 1 080 817, 60.8%) of amenable deaths in newborns were attributable to poor quality care rather than lack of access to care [25]. The current effort to achieve the Sustainable Development Goals will require more robust attention to the quality of care provided, as well as to improvements in how these services are measured [18,26].

Current global measurement focuses on crude coverage indicators such as whether or not a woman received any antenatal care or whether or not a skilled birth attendant was present at delivery, measures which are self-reported through household surveys [19]. Effective coverage is a metric that unites need, use, and quality to more reliably capture the relationship between health service delivery and population health outcomes [27,28]. Current literature uses a range of quality measures – including measures of structure [29,30], process of care [31,32], and health outcomes [33] – to calculate effective coverage or quality-adjusted coverage. The specific focus of our analysis is adjusting crude maternal care coverage for measures of nutrition intervention content and quality. Adjusting coverage estimates for the quality of care provided can yield greater insight into health system performance and potential population health benefits of accessing care. However, the data on valid quality measures are sparse and more challenging to obtain than self-reported health care utilization measures: household surveys address content of care inconsistently [34], and maternal recall of specific interventions is highly variable by intervention, context, and survey timing [35-37]. Given the known benefit of maternal nutrition intervention on neonatal outcomes such as birthweight and breastfeeding, we use health system and population information to define nutrition quality-adjusted coverage metrics and quantify their impact on breastfeeding and birthweight.

METHODS

We used household survey data to generate estimates of health care utilization among those in need (crude coverage), and health facility clinical observation data to summarize the content of care provided in the service environment accessible to each woman. We linked crude coverage and service environment information to adjust individual-level coverage metrics for quality of nutrition interventions. Malawi was used as the case study for testing this approach due to the country's success in achieving the MDG child mortality target, the high utilization of maternal health care, and the availability of both population and health facility data [38].

Data sources and study sample

Data on women with recent births or young children were obtained from the 2013-2014 Malawi Multiple Indicator Cluster Survey (MICS), a nationally representative survey conducted in collaboration between the Malawi government and the United Nations Children's Fund (UNICEF). Households were selected from previously defined enumeration areas (EAs) based on the 2008 census. Of 25 430 eligible women aged 15-49, 24 230 were successfully interviewed (95.3% response rate). We extracted information on household, maternal, and child characteristics for live births in the preceding two years. We obtained the exact spatial location of EA centroids from the Malawi National Statistical Office in order to link the EA location with health facilities providing antenatal and delivery care.

Data on health facilities and services were obtained from the 2013 Malawi Service Provision Assessment (SPA), a census of formal-sector health facilities conducted by the Demographic and Health Surveys (DHS) program. Geospatial coordinates were collected for all facilities, as were urban vs rural location, district, and region name. We divided facilities based on district and urban location to match the 31 districts and cities included in the MICS.

For facilities providing ANC, with or without delivery care, the SPA survey team conducted direct observation of ANC visits and interviews with women following ANC. Visits were sampled for inclusion using systematic random sampling based on the number of clients present during the day of the assessment, with a goal of sampling a maximum of five visits per provider and fifteen per facility. Interviewers attempted to oversample first ANC visits if possible; for this analysis, ANC visits were defined as first, second, third, fourth or later based on client report. The survey team attempted to complete a direct observation of normal delivery at facilities providing normal delivery care. Observations for either ANC or delivery could not be conducted if services were available on the day of the assessment, but no clients presented for care.

Infant and child outcomes

We defined two outcomes that should be affected by nutritional interventions during ANC for which data are available from the MICS questionnaire: birth-weight and immediate breastfeeding.

Infant birthweight in kilograms was defined from maternal recall; the survey team verified weight from infant health cards where available. In keeping with prior analyses, we used multiple imputation to estimate birthweight for missing values [39]; we used a linear regression model using covariates of child size (categorical, based on maternal recall), neonatal death and male sex as well as the exposures and covariates of the analytic model defined below and generated 5 imputed data sets. Low birthweight was defined as birthweight less than or equal to 2.5 kg. Birthweight analysis was restricted to singleton births; each delivery resulting in multiple children was included as a single observation for the analysis of immediate breastfeeding.

Immediate breastfeeding was defined based on maternal report of putting the infant to breast within 1 hour of birth.

Crude coverage

Crude ANC coverage was defined based on women's self-reported number of ANC visits in the MICS. Intrapartum care coverage was defined as self-report of childbirth at a formal health facility.

Quality of nutrition interventions at health facilities

We used direct observation of ANC and delivery care from the SPA to estimate how frequently facilities provided evidence-based nutrition interventions.

We identified three nutrition interventions that should be delivered during ANC: provision of iron-folic acid (IFA) supplements and counseling on their side effects, counseling on appropriate nutrition and diets during pregnancy, and counseling and support for early and exclusive breastfeeding (the direct observation protocol in the SPA does not provide a specific time period such as within 1 hour for the content of counseling on early breastfeeding). Each ANC observation was scored from 0 to 1 on each of these three interventions; we calculated provision of each intervention at the facility level by averaging scores across observations with the same visit number (first visit, second visit, etc.). We also calculated average adherence at the district level and imputed missing facility values with the district average when a facility had no visits of a particular number or no visits at all observed. We added up expected interventions across visit numbers for each facility to calculate the number of times a woman seeking ANC for a given number of visits at that facility could expect to receive each evidence-based nutrition intervention.

Similarly, we identified post-delivery interventions to improve breastfeeding uptake. The primary measure of interest was direct observation of breastfeeding initiation within 1 hour of delivery. We defined a secondary measure based on observation of breastfeeding initiation, the newborn being placed skin-to-skin if breathing, and keeping the mother and newborn in the same room. Each delivery observation was scored as 0 or 1 for immediate breastfeeding and then from 0 to 1 based on performance of these three actions. Facility scores were calculated as the average score across observations.

Calculation of adjusted coverage: Antenatal care

The MICS does not provide information on the type of health facility where women sought ANC or other details that would enable matching women to a specific facility. We therefore calculated intervention provision based on the health service environment for each EA. The national health policy of Malawi defines 8 km as the maximum acceptable distance to a facility providing the essential health package (including reproductive health care); we therefore defined the health service environment for ANC as the health facilities providing ANC services within 8 km of the patient's EA, or the single nearest ANC facility if none are within that distance. In urban areas with many health facilities, we limited the service environment to 5 km due to the large number of facilities available to women.

We averaged expected intervention provision scores per number of ANC visits across the service environment, weighting facilities by the ANC patient volume on the day of the visit to reflect greater use of larger facilities, like hospitals, than less busy clinics. We averaged service environment quality scores for IFA and ANC nutrition counseling to capture health system contributions to birthweight for a given number of ANC visits, and we averaged cumulative scores for nutrition counseling and breastfeeding support as inputs contributing to breastfeeding outcomes. These scores capture the expected provision of nutrition interventions for a given number of ANC visits in a specific geographic area.

Each woman in the MICS with a live birth in the past 2 years was assigned the adjusted coverage score corresponding to the number of ANC visits she reported. Quality-adjusted coverage scores could range from 0 (no ANC or no interventions delivered) to the number of ANC visits received (all interventions delivered at all visits), with women reporting four or more visits assigned the same score.

Calculation of adjusted coverage: Post-delivery care

Childbirth services are offered at 540 health facilities in Malawi, but at 318 facilities no women gave birth on the day of the SPA visit, leaving 222 facilities with at least one directly observed delivery for analysis. We therefore calculated quality-adjusted coverage of post-delivery nutrition interventions at the district (as opposed to EA) level. We averaged the facility scores for these interventions by district, stratified by hospital or non-hospital facility type. We imputed regional averages by facility tier for 3 missing observations (2 districts with no hospitals with a delivery observation, 1 district with no non-hospitals with a delivery observation). We assigned each woman from the MICS with a live birth in the past 2 years an adjusted coverage score based on her reported delivery facility type and district of residence; these scores capture likelihood of receipt of post-delivery intervention based on geographic area and delivery facility type. Women delivering outside of the formal health system were scored as 0.

Covariates

We extracted household and maternal characteristics from the MICS data, including rural location, household wealth quintile based on an asset index, maternal education (none, primary, secondary and above), maternal age, parity, and birth spacing in months. We calculated the square of maternal age to account for nonlinear associations between maternal age and infant outcomes. Birth interval is set to zero for first births.

Statistical analysis

To account for missing data due to incomplete MICS responses (aside from birthweight) or lack of spatial coordinates for the EA, we calculated inverse probability weights for each individual-level outcome. We fit logistic regression models with the outcome of complete data and covariates of quality-adjusted coverage, household wealth index, maternal age, primiparity, and birth spacing and predicted the probability each observation was complete. For complete observations, we calculated the inverse probability of being observed to up-weight observations most similar to the missing cases. This method relies on the assumption of missing at random: that the missing cases are exchangeable with the observed cases conditional on the observed covariates. We rescaled weights to match the analytic sample size and, for descriptive analysis, multiplied the inverse probability weight with the MICS survey sampling weight. For adjusted analysis, we used only the inverse probability weight.

We present descriptive statistics of the sample of recent singleton births, including proportions for binary and categorical variables and median and IQR for continuous variables; all analyses are weighted to account for missing data and sample design. We describe the frequency of interventions during ANC using the individual direct observations of care, weighted with the SPA survey sampling weight. We map median levels of crude and quality-adjusted coverage during ANC at the district level for illustration.

In adjusted analysis, we fit generalized linear models with a log link to estimate the relative risk of low birthweight associated with first crude coverage and then quality-adjusted coverage of nutrition interventions. Models are adjusted for rural location, household wealth quintile, maternal age, maternal age squared, maternal education, birth spacing, and first child. Models for low birthweight account for the variance introduced by multiple imputation. We fit the same models with the outcome of immediate breastfeeding and test the exposures of crude coverage (number of ANC visits, facility delivery) and quality-adjusted coverage of breastfeeding-related interventions during ANC and intrapartum care. These models are weighted to account for missing data and provide clustered standard errors due to repeated sampling within EAs.

Ethical approval

The original survey implementers obtained ethical approvals for data collection; the Harvard University Research Protection Program deemed this analysis exempt from human subjects review.

RESULTS

Content and quality of nutrition interventions

Of the 1060 facilities on a master list maintained by the Ministry of Health at the time of the SPA survey, 83 were closed, inaccessible, or refused assessment; 977 facilities were successfully assessed (92%), of which 643 provided ANC services and 540 provided normal delivery care. A total of 2068 ANC visits and 474 normal deliveries were directly observed, yielding a median of 5 ANC observations and 1 delivery observation per facility.

Figure 1 shows the delivery of nutrition interventions during directly observed ANC visits. Only 10% of women in the first through third visit and 5% in fourth or later visits had IFA prescribed with appropriate counseling; between 80%

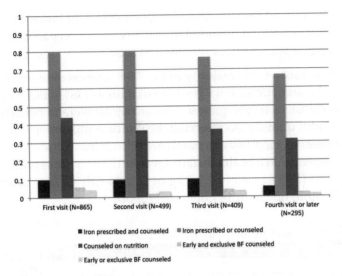

Figure 1. *Delivery of nutrition-related interventions during ANC visits (N = 2068 directly observed visits). ANC – antenatal care, BF – breastfeeding.*

(first visit) and 67% (fourth or later visit) of women received an iron prescription alone or counseling without prescription. Counseling on appropriate nutrition during pregnancy was observed in 44% of first visits but only 32% of fourth or later visits. Counseling on early or exclusive breastfeeding was rarely observed: during first visits, only 5.7% of women were counseled on early and on exclusive breastfeeding and 4.2% were counseled on one of these, with even lower frequencies in later visits.

Across the 474 observed deliveries, 90.6% of mothers were seen to initiate breastfeeding within an hour of delivery, 78.9% of newborns were placed directly skin-to-skin, and 91.3% of mother-newborn dyads were kept in the same room following delivery.

Coverage of maternal care

The MICS sample included 7576 women with a live birth in the past two years, including 173 women delivering twins. We excluded 104 women living in EAs with undefined location, 76 who did not report a specific number of ANC visits, 1 with no information on educational attainment, and 10 cases of multiple births without valid time of breastfeeding initiation. The remaining 7385 observations were eligible for one or both analyses (birthweight and/or breastfeeding). The analysis for which birthweight was the outcome included 7225 singleton live births (97.6% of singleton births in the sample), 6123 (84.7%) of which had birthweight reported based on a health card or maternal recall. The immediate breastfeeding analysis included 7235 live births with valid self-reported time of breastfeeding initiation (95.5% of births in the sample); a single observation was included for each twin delivery as maternal report of breastfeeding was constant within twin sets.

As shown in **Table 1**, the majority of the 7385 women delivering in the past 2 years in the analytic sample lived in rural areas (88%) and had a primary education (71%). Nearly a quarter of recent births were in households in the poorest wealth quintile. As expected, health care utilization was high, with 98% of women seeking any antenatal care (45% at least four visits) and 91% of children delivered in a health facility. Of the 6123 newborns with birthweight reported, 933 (15.5%) weighed 2.5 kg or less. Nearly 80% of newborns were breastfed within one hour per maternal report.

Table 1. *Characteristics of live births past 2 y (N = 7385)*

	N	%
Rural	6510	88.2%
Maternal education:		
None	855	11.6%
Primary	5241	71.0%
Secondary and above	1289	17.5%
Household wealth quintile:		
1 (Poorest)	1824	24.7%
2	1653	22.4%
3	1536	20.8%
4	1230	16.7%
5 (Wealthiest)	1142	15.5%
First child to this mother	1666	22.6%
Child delivered in health facility	6705	90.8%
Mother attended any antenatal care visits	7218	97.7%
Mother attended at least 4 ANC visits	3333	45.1%
Low birth weight (N = 6123)	933	15.5%
Breastfed immediately (N = 7235)	5628	77.8%
	MEDIAN	**IQR**
Birth spacing (months, if not first child, N = 5534)	40	31-55
Maternal age at birth (years)	25.5	20.8-30.8
Number of times mother attended ANC	3	3-4
Iron-folate interventions in ANC	1.59	1.22-1.99
Nutrition counseling in ANC	1.01	0.57-1.68
Breastfeeding counseling in ANC	0.06	0.00-0.20
Composite birthweight-related interventions in ANC (iron-folate and nutrition)	1.36	1.00-1.79
Composite breastfeeding-related interventions in ANC (breastfeeding counseling and nutrition)	0.57	0.33-0.97
Facility delivery with immediate breastfeeding	1.00	0.79–1.00
Facility delivery with breastfeeding interventions (immediate breastfeeding, rooming in, skin to skin)	0.88	0.67-0.97

ANC – antenatal care, IQR – interquartile range

Crude and adjusted coverage of ANC

After adjustment for nutrition-related quality of ANC in the service environment, women received nutrition interventions considerably less often than they sought care: over the course of ANC women attended a median of 3 ANC visits but received a median of 1.6 interventions on IFA (either prescriptions for supplements or counseling on IFA adherence and side effects with and without IFA), 1 instance of counseling on diet during pregnancy, and 0.06 instances of counseling on optimal breastfeeding. Women thus received a median of 1.35 maternal nutrition interventions and 0.57 interventions that might increase uptake of breastfeeding.

Figure 2 provides a geographic summary of crude ANC coverage and coverage adjusted for receipt of nutrition interventions and breastfeeding interventions at the district level. Women accessed ANC at high levels across the country (**Figure 2**, panel A). Despite this utilization, women were receiving relatively few nutrition interventions that can improve infant birthweight (**Figure 2**, panel B) or improve breastfeeding uptake (**Figure 2**, panel C). Because coverage of nutrition interventions varies, access to ANC does not directly correspond to complete care. For instance, within the Northern Region, Karonga district bordering Lake Malawi had a median of 3 ANC visits per woman (average

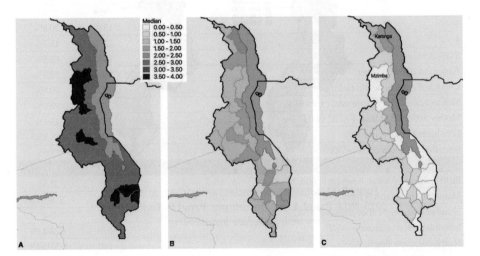

Figure 2. *Nutrition interventions during ANC in Malawi, 2013 – 2014.* **Panel A.** *ANC utilization: Median ANC visits among women with live singleton birth in past 2 years by district.* **Panel B.** *Nutrition interventions: Median interventions related to maternal nutrition (IFA, nutrition counseling) during ANC visits among women with live singleton birth in past 2 years by district.* **Panel C.** *Breastfeeding interventions: Median interventions related to breastfeeding (maternal nutrition counseling, breastfeeding counseling) during ANC visits among women with live singleton birth in past 2 years by district. ANC – antenatal care, IFA – iron-folic acid.*

of 3.4) but provides a median of 2.4 maternal nutrition interventions within those visits and 1.5 breastfeeding interventions, the highest in the country. In contrast, nearby Mzimba district had 4 median ANC visits but only 1.2 maternal nutrition interventions and 0.4 breastfeeding interventions; inferring receipt of nutrition-related interventions from crude ANC coverage can lead to erroneous conclusions. In all districts, the number of ANC visits exceeded the provision of essential nutrition interventions.

Crude and adjusted coverage of delivery care

Figure 3 provides a geographic summary of delivery coverage and coverage adjusted for immediate breastfeeding at the district level, again showing high levels of health service utilization in panel A. While a few districts showed drops between facility delivery and delivery with observed immediate breastfeeding (**Figure 3**, panel B), many districts achieved high coverage and high adjusted coverage.

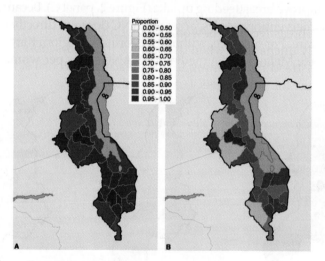

Figure 3. *Nutritional interventions at childbirth in Malawi, 2013-2014.* **Panel A.** *Facility delivery.* **Panel B.** *Facility delivery with immediate breastfeeding.*

Association of coverage with health outcomes

Both crude and quality-adjusted ANC coverage were associated with lower risk of low birthweight newborns in multivariable regression (**Table 2**, panel A). The risk of a low birthweight newborn is 10% lower with each additional ANC visit and 13% lower with each additional nutrition-related intervention (adjusted relative risk (ARR) = 0.87, 95% confidence interval (CI) = 0.79, 0.96).

These models suggest that if women received all of the recommended nutrition interventions at each ANC visit they currently attend, the population prevalence of low birthweight would decrease by almost 3 percentage points, from 13.7% (95% CI = 13.6, 13.8) to an estimated 10.8% (95% CI = 10.7, 10.9).

Crude and adjusted coverage of ANC and delivery are also associated with greater likelihood of immediate breastfeeding in models adjusted for demographic and individual characteristics (**Table 2**, panel B). Nutrition quality-adjusted measures show slightly stronger links: the likelihood of initiating breastfeeding immediately is 4% higher with each additional breastfeeding intervention received during ANC (ARR = 1.04, 95% CI = 1.02, 1.07) and 8% higher for facility delivery with breastfeeding interventions compared to women without quality care at delivery (ARR = 1.08, 95% CI = 1.02, 1.14). This suggests that the population prevalence of immediate breastfeeding would increase from 75.9% (95% CI = 75.8, 76.0) to 86.0% (95% CI = 85.8, 86.1) if women received nutrition-related interventions in their current ANC visits and facility delivery; almost all of this potential increase (9.7 percentage points) is attributed to increased quality of ANC given the already high prevalence of immediate breastfeeding for women delivering in health facilities. Results are essentially unchanged when using three indicators (observation of immediate breastfeeding, rooming in, and placing newborn skin to skin) to adjust coverage for post-delivery care (not shown).

Table 2. *Association of coverage and quality-adjusted coverage with newborn health outcomes*

	ADJUSTED RELATIVE RISK	95% CONFIDENCE INTERVAL
A: Low birthweight (N = 7225):		
Model A1:*		
Number of ANC† visits	0.90	0.85, 0.95
Model A2:*		
Number of nutrition-related interventions in ANC	0.87	0.79, 0.96
B: Immediate breastfeeding (N = 7235):		
Model B1:*		
Number of ANC visits	1.01	1.00, 1.02
Facility delivery	1.06	1.00, 1.13
Model B2:*		
Number of breastfeeding-related interventions in ANC	1.04	1.02, 1.07
Facility delivery with immediate breastfeeding	1.08	1.02, 1.14

ANC – antenatal care

*All models are controlled for: rural/urban location, maternal age at birth and age squared, wealth quintile, maternal education (none, primary, secondary or greater), first birth, birth spacing (months). Models are weighted to account for observations excluded due to missing data; confidence intervals account for clustering due to repeated samples within enumeration area. Models with low birthweight as an outcome are based on 5 data sets with multiple imputation for missing birthweight.

DISCUSSION

In low and middle-income countries, one in four neonatal deaths occur in low birthweight infants [40,41]. Maternal nutrition supplementation and counseling during ANC and support for immediate initiation of breastfeeding after delivery are important interventions for improving birthweight and reducing neonatal mortality. Household surveys do not consistently and reliably capture data on coverage of these interventions [34,42], and reported crude coverage estimates, such as number of ANC visits or facility delivery, do not capture the content of these services or their quality.

In this study, we applied a method for incorporating nutrition interventions into coverage estimates of ANC and post-delivery care by linking observed data from health facility service provision assessments to self-reported health care utilization from household surveys. These individual-level adjusted coverage metrics were associated with lower risk of low birthweight newborns and higher probability of immediate breastfeeding, demonstrating their salience to population health outcomes. An additional ANC visit including nutritional interventions was associated with a 13% lower risk of low birthweight compared to a 10% reduction for an additional ANC visit without considering nutrition interventions. Based on these models, if women were to receive all recommended nutrition interventions during antenatal care, population prevalence of low birth weight would decrease by an estimated 3 percentage points, from 14% to 11%. If effected, this 21% relative reduction in low birth weight could reduce neonatal mortality at a population level.

Nutrition-adjusted coverage interventions for both ANC and post-delivery care were also associated with greater likelihood that mothers will initiate breastfeeding within 1 hour of birth. The likelihood of initiating immediate breastfeeding was 4% higher with each additional breastfeeding intervention received during ANC and 8% higher for delivery in a facility with breastfeeding interventions. Ensuring breastfeeding-related interventions are delivered as intended within existing ANC and delivery care could lead to an estimated 10% increase (76% to 86%) in the prevalence of immediately breastfed infants, largely driven by potential improvements in the content of ANC. Immediate breastfeeding is associated with substantial mortality reductions in all infants and among those exclusively breastfed [7]; an increase in population rates of immediate breastfeeding can contribute to newborn survival [43].

Findings from this study suggest substantial population health benefits from a focus on health care quality given the high levels of utilization already achieved. This expands on prior work evaluating access and quality of care in Malawi [31,44] and underscores the government's emphasis on quality improvement as a health sector priority, particularly within the Maternal-Neonatal Health section [45-47]. While the gap between utilization and quality (provision of evidence-based interventions) is notable in Malawi, other studies have documented deficits in care content for ANC even when utilization is high [29,34,48-51]. Self-reported 90-day coverage of iron for pregnant women was 33% in 2015-2016 [52]; while women may obtain iron outside the formal health sector or without prompting from a clinician, the deficit even in self-reported coverage supports our finding of missed opportunities to improve health. Scalable strategies to increase intervention delivery are needed to address these gaps. For example, while stock outs of iron folate could shape provider behaviors on prescribing and counseling, breastfeeding promotion, which was done rarely by health providers in this study, does not require intensive resources, can be delivered at all levels of the health system and can be performed by competent health workers or in the group setting at any ANC visit [53].

Quality-adjusted and effective coverage metrics for maternal, newborn, and child health and nutrition are necessary to benchmark and guide the type of health system strengthening that can result in better population health by addressing both access and quality [18,19,54]. Development of valid and reliable metrics has been limited to date due to the reliance on household surveys. Self-reported measures of content of care may be unreliable when recall pertains to services or advice rendered during labor and delivery, when recall periods are prolonged, or when care pertains to socially desirable behaviors [35,36,42]. This study is the first to develop and apply nutrition-related metrics of effective coverage for antenatal and labor care and to demonstrate the relevance of such metrics for population health outcomes. It employs a novel methodology of calculating quality-adjusted coverage at the individual and population level by combining health facility and population assessments using exact geographic information and employing direct observation of care to provide reliable estimates of delivery of nutrition interventions. The results underscore the importance of delivering these interventions with quality to improve maternal and neonatal outcomes.

From a measurement perspective, this study was possible due to the contemporaneous SPA and MICS surveys in Malawi and the availability of geographic information to link them. Relatively few instances of overlapping surveys exist to date. Data from health facility assessments such as the SPA are under-utilized, and there are far fewer of these surveys than DHS and MICS. To make the best use of these data sources, there is a need to coordinate the data collected [55], both at a broad scale of survey timing and locations as well as at a granular level in collecting more details on household surveys regarding type of facility used and whether it is the closest facility of that type to enable closer linking. Efforts to align health facility surveys such as the SPA, Service Delivery Indicators, and Service Availability and Readiness Assessment to provide a common basis for content of care assessment are an important step [56]. Ongoing monitoring of effective coverage will demand fresh thinking around incorporating routine data sources, such as linking detailed quality information like the SPA to sparser but more frequently measured elements such as health management information systems (HMIS). Further research on methods to enhance and make use of routine data collection is warranted.

There are several important limitations to our study. One of the primary outcomes was birthweight: we imputed birthweight for 15% of the observations due to missing data, relying on the assumptions that the data were missing at random and that the imputation model was correctly specified. A novel aspect of this work is our approach to linked health service provision data and household survey information in order to come up with quality adjusted metrics for individual women. Our data sources were not exactly contemporaneous – the MICS was carried out in 2013-2014 and the SPA was done in 2013. Due to the recall period for live birth, ANC visits may have taken place up to 2 years and 9 months before the survey; recall may be imperfect and quality of care may vary across this time period. We were not able to explicitly link mothers to specific facilities based on available data and relied on average quality across the nearby service environment; estimates of delivery care quality were based on observations of deliveries during the facility assessment, meaning less information is available on low-volume facilities than high-volume facilities. Finally, given the observational data, residual confounding due to unmeasured variables may bias the results.

Our findings show it is feasible to combine health facility and population data to incorporate quality into crude coverage measures in order to address the coverage and quality of nutrition interventions as part of antenatal, delivery, and newborn care. The findings are in line with results from clinical studies that demonstrate health impact of nutrition interventions on breastfeeding practices and low birth weight [53,57]. The results show that quality-adjusted measures demonstrate clear links to individual health outcomes of global health importance, supporting their utility for health system assessment. These findings also suggest that improvements in quality may have the potential to reduce neonatal mortality in Malawi within the existing high levels of health system coverage.

Acknowledgements: *The authors thank Humphreys Nsona for assistance in obtaining geospatial information. The members of the the Countdown 2030 Coverage Technical Working Group are: Agbessi Amouzou, Shams El Arifeen, Ties Boerma, Robert Black, Liliana Carvajal-Valez, Doris Chou, Shelley Walton, Chika Hayashi, Safia Jiwani, Sennen Hounton, Margaret E Kruk, Hannah H Leslie, Mengija Liang, Honorati Masanja, Purnima Menon, Allisyn Moran, Lois Park, Jennifer Requejo, Lara ME Vaz, and Bill Weiss.*

Ethical approval: *The original survey implementers obtained ethical approvals for data collection; the Harvard University Research Protection Program deemed this analysis exempt from human subjects review.*

Funding: *This work was supported by a grant of the Bill & Melinda Gates Foundation to the Countdown to 2030 for Women's, Children's and Adolescents' Health (OPP114893), through US Fund for UNICEF.*

Authorship contributions: *Initial conceptualization: NTJ, HHL. Refining study design: EP, DL, AM. Data management: DL, HHL. Analysis: NTJ, DL, HHL. First draft: NTJ, HHL. Critical revision: EP, DL, AM.*

Competing interests: *The authors completed the Unified Competing Interest form at www. icmje.org/coi_disclosure.pdf (available upon request from the corresponding author). Dr Piwoz reports being an employee of the Bill & Melinda Gates Foundation during the conduct of the study; Mr Lee and Dr Leslie report grant support from the Bill & Melinda Gates Foundation during the conduct of the study. The authors declare no other conflicts of interest.*

References

1 Smith ER, Shankar AH, Wu LS, Aboud S, Adu-Afarwuah S, Ali H, et al. Modifiers of the effect of maternal multiple micronutrient supplementation on stillbirth, birth outcomes, and infant mortality: a meta-analysis of individual patient data from 17 randomised trials in low-income and middle-income countries. Lancet Glob Health. 2017;5:e1090-100. Medline:29025632 doi:10.1016/S2214-109X(17)30371-6

2 Liu L, Oza S, Hogan D, Chu Y, Perin J, Zhu J, et al. Global, regional, and national causes of under-5 mortality in 2000-15: an updated systematic analysis with implications for the Sustainable Development Goals. Lancet. 2016;388:3027-35. Medline:27839855 doi:10.1016/S0140-6736(16)31593-8

3 Bhutta ZA, Das JK, Rizvi A, Gaffey MF, Walker N, Horton S, et al. Evidence-based interventions for improvement of maternal and child nutrition: what can be done and at what cost? Lancet. 2013;382:452-77. Medline:23746776 doi:10.1016/S0140-6736(13)60996-4

4 Caulfield LE, de Onis M, Blossner M, Black RE. Undernutrition as an underlying cause of child deaths associated with diarrhea, pneumonia, malaria, and measles. Am J Clin Nutr. 2004;80:193-8. Medline:15213048 doi:10.1093/ajcn/80.1.193

5 UNICEF. The State of the World's Children 2006. New York: UNICEF, 2005.

6 Bhutta ZA, Das JK. Interventions to address maternal and childhood undernutrition: current evidence. Nestle Nutr Inst Workshop Ser. 2014;78:59-69. Medline:24504207 doi:10.1159/000354941

7 Smith ER, Hurt L, Chowdhury R, Sinha B, Fawzi W, Edmond KM, et al. Delayed breastfeeding initiation and infant survival: A systematic review and meta-analysis. PLoS One. 2017;12:e0180722. Medline:28746353 doi:10.1371/journal.pone.0180722

8 Lawn JE, Blencowe H, Oza S, You D, Lee AC, Waiswa P, et al. Every Newborn: progress, priorities, and potential beyond survival. Lancet. 2014;384:189-205. Medline:24853593 doi:10.1016/S0140-6736(14)60496-7

9 Black RE, Allen LH, Bhutta ZA, Caulfield LE, de Onis M, Ezzati M, et al. Maternal and child undernutrition: global and regional exposures and health consequences. Lancet. 2008;371:243-60. Medline:18207566 doi:10.1016/S0140-6736(07)61690-0

10 Smith ER, Locks LM, Manji KP, McDonald CM, Kupka R, Kisenge R, et al. Delayed breastfeeding initiation is associated with infant morbidity. J Pediatr. 2017;191:57-62. e2. Medline:29173323 doi:10.1016/j.jpeds.2017.08.069

11 Victora CG, Bahl R, Barros AJD, França GVA, Horton S, Krasevec J, et al. Breastfeeding in the 21st century: epidemiology, mechanisms, and lifelong effect. Lancet. 2016;387:475-90. Medline:26869575 doi:10.1016/S0140-6736(15)01024-7

12   Christian P, Mullany LC, Hurley KM, Katz J, Black RE. Nutrition and maternal, neonatal, and child health. Semin Perinatol. 2015;39:361-72. Medline:26166560 doi:10.1053/j.semperi.2015.06.009

13   Grummer-Strawn LM, Rollins N. Summarising the health effects of breastfeeding. Acta Paediatrica. 2015;104:1-2. Medline:26535930 doi:10.1111/apa.13136

14   Horta BL, Loret de Mola C, Victora CG. Long-term consequences of breastfeeding on cholesterol, obesity, systolic blood pressure and type 2 diabetes: a systematic review and meta-analysis. Acta Paediatr. 2015;104:30-7. Medline:26192560 doi:10.1111/apa.13133

15   World Health Organization. WHO recommendations on antenatal care for a positive pregnancy experience. Geneva, Switzerland: World Health Organization, 2016.

16   Kuhnt J, Vollmer S. Antenatal care services and its implications for vital and health outcomes of children: evidence from 193 surveys in 69 low-income and middle-income countries. BMJ Open. 2017;7:e017122. Medline:29146636 doi:10.1136/bmjopen-2017-017122

17   Victora CG, Requejo JH, Barros AJ, Berman P, Bhutta Z, Boerma T, et al. Countdown to 2015: a decade of tracking progress for maternal, newborn, and child survival. Lancet. 2016;387:2049-59. Medline:26477328 doi:10.1016/S0140-6736(15)00519-X

18   Kruk ME, Gage A, Arsenault C, Jordan K, Leslie H, Roder-DeWan S, et al. High quality health systems—time for a revolution: Report of the Lancet Global Health Commission on High Quality Health Systems in the SDG Era. Lancet Glob Health. 2018;6:e1196-252. Medline:30196093 doi:10.1016/S2214-109X(18)30386-3

19   Countdown to 2030 Collaboration. Countdown to 2030: tracking progress towards universal coverage for reproductive, maternal, newborn, and child health. Lancet. 2018;391:1538-48. Medline:29395268 doi:10.1016/S0140-6736(18)30104-1

20   Chari AV., Okeke EN Can institutional deliveries reduce newborn mortality? Evidence from Rwanda. RAND Working Paper. 2014; WR 1072. Available: https://www.rand.org/pubs/working_papers/WR1072.html. Accessed: 10 January 2020.

21   Abou-Zahr CL, Wardlaw TM. Antenatal care in developing countries: promises, achievements and missed opportunities: an analysis of trends, levels and differentials, 1990-2001. Geneva: WHO; 2003.

22   Benova L, Tunçalp Ö, Moran AC, Campbell OMR. Not just a number: examining coverage and content of antenatal care in low-income and middle-income countries. BMJ Glob Health. 2018;3:e000779. Medline:29662698 doi:10.1136/bmjgh-2018-000779

23   de Onis M, Dewey KG, Borghi E, Onyango AW, Blossner M, Daelmans B, et al. The World Health Organization's global target for reducing childhood stunting by 2025: rationale and proposed actions. Matern Child Nutr. 2013;9 Suppl 2:6-26. Medline:24074315 doi:10.1111/mcn.12075

24   Imdad A, Yakoob MY, Bhutta ZA. Effect of breastfeeding promotion interventions on breastfeeding rates, with special focus on developing countries. BMC Public Health. 2011;11:S24. Medline:21501442 doi:10.1186/1471-2458-11-S3-S24

25   Kruk ME, Gage AD, Joseph NT, Danaei G, García-Saisó S, Salomon JA. Mortality due to low-quality health systems in the universal health coverage era: a systematic analysis of amenable deaths in 137 countries. Lancet. 2018;392:2203-12. Medline:30195398 doi:10.1016/S0140-6736(18)31668-4

26   Sobel HL, Huntington D, Temmerman M. Quality at the centre of universal health coverage. Health Policy Plan. 2016;31:547-9. Medline:26420642 doi:10.1093/heapol/czv095

27   Ng M, Fullman N, Dieleman JL, Flaxman AD, Murray CJL, Lim SS. Effective Coverage: A Metric for Monitoring Universal Health Coverage. PLoS Med. 2014;11:e1001730. Medline:25243780 doi:10.1371/journal.pmed.1001730

28 Boerma T, AbouZahr C, Evans D, Evans T. Monitoring Intervention Coverage in the Context of Universal Health Coverage. PLoS Med. 2014;11:e1001728. Medline:25243586 doi:10.1371/journal.pmed.1001728

29 Baker U, Okuga M, Waiswa P, Manzi F, Peterson S, Hanson C. Bottlenecks in the implementation of essential screening tests in antenatal care: Syphilis, HIV, and anemia testing in rural Tanzania and Uganda. Int J Gynaecol Obstet. 2015;130:S43-50. Medline:26054252 doi:10.1016/j.ijgo.2015.04.017

30 Baker U, Peterson S, Marchant T, Mbaruku G, Temu S, Manzi F, et al. Identifying implementation bottlenecks for maternal and newborn health interventions in rural districts of the United Republic of Tanzania. Bull World Health Organ. 2015;93:380-9. Medline:26240459 doi:10.2471/BLT.14.141879

31 Leslie HH, Malata A, Ndiaye Y, Kruk ME. Effective coverage of primary care services in eight high-mortality countries. BMJ Glob Health. 2017;2:e000424. Medline:29632704 doi:10.1136/bmjgh-2017-000424

32 Marchant T, Tilley-Gyado RD, Tessema T, Singh K, Gautham M, Umar N, et al. Adding Content to Contacts: Measurement of High Quality Contacts for Maternal and Newborn Health in Ethiopia, North East Nigeria, and Uttar Pradesh, India. PLoS One. 2015;10:e0126840. Medline:26000829 doi:10.1371/journal.pone.0126840

33 Colson KE, Zúñiga-Brenes P, Ríos-Zertuche D, Conde-Glez CJ, Gagnier MC, Palmisano E, et al. Comparative Estimates of Crude and Effective Coverage of Measles Immunization in Low-Resource Settings: Findings from Salud Mesoamérica 2015. PLoS One. 2015;10:e0130697. Medline:26136239 doi:10.1371/journal.pone.0130697

34 Arsenault C, Jordan K, Lee D, Dinsa G, Manzi F, Marchant T, et al. Equity in antenatal care quality: an analysis of 91 national household surveys. Lancet Glob Health. 2018;6:e1186-95. Medline:30322649 doi:10.1016/S2214-109X(18)30389-9

35 Blanc AK, Diaz C, McCarthy KJ, Berdichevsky K. Measuring progress in maternal and newborn health care in Mexico: validating indicators of health system contact and quality of care. BMC Pregnancy Childbirth. 2016;16:255. Medline:27577266 doi:10.1186/s12884-016-1047-0

36 McCarthy KJ, Blanc AK, Warren CE, Kimani J, Mdawida B, Ndwidga C. Can surveys of women accurately track indicators of maternal and newborn care? A validity and reliability study in Kenya. J Glob Health. 2016;6:020502. Medline:27606061 doi:10.7189/jogh.06.020502

37 Bryce J, Arnold F, Blanc A, Hancioglu A, Newby H, Requejo J, et al. Measuring coverage in MNCH: new findings, new strategies, and recommendations for action. PLoS Med. 2013;10:e1001423. Medline:23667340 doi:10.1371/journal.pmed.1001423

38 Doherty T, Zembe W, Ngandu N, Kinney M, Manda S, Besada D, et al. Assessment of Malawi's success in child mortality reduction through the lens of the Catalytic Initiative Integrated Health Systems Strengthening programme: Retrospective evaluation. J Glob Health. 2015;5:020412. Medline:26649176 doi:10.7189/jogh.05.020412

39 Katz J, Lee AC, Kozuki N, Lawn JE, Cousens S, Blencowe H, et al. Mortality risk in preterm and small-for-gestational-age infants in low-income and middle-income countries: a pooled country analysis. Lancet. 2013;382:417-25. Medline:23746775 doi:10.1016/S0140-6736(13)60993-9

40 Lawn JE, Cousens S, Zupan J. 4 million neonatal deaths: when? Where? Why? Lancet. 2005;365:891-900. Medline:15752534 doi:10.1016/S0140-6736(05)71048-5

41 Lee AC, Kozuki N, Cousens S, Stevens GA, Blencowe H, Silveira MF, et al. Estimates of burden and consequences of infants born small for gestational age in low and middle income countries with INTERGROWTH-21(st) standard: analysis of CHERG datasets. BMJ. 2017;358:j3677. Medline:28819030 doi:10.1136/bmj.j3677

42 Bryce J, Arnold F, Blanc A, Hancioglu A, Newby H, Requejo J, et al. Measuring coverage in MNCH: new findings, new strategies, and recommendations for action. PLoS Med. 2013;10:e1001423. Medline:23667340 doi:10.1371/journal.pmed.1001423

43 Sankar MJ, Sinha B, Chowdhury R, Bhandari N, Taneja S, Martines J, et al. Optimal breastfeeding practices and infant and child mortality: a systematic review and meta-analysis. Acta Paediatrica. 2015;104:3-13. Medline:26249674 doi:10.1111/apa.13147

44 Leslie HH, Fink G, Nsona H, Kruk ME. Obstetric Facility Quality and Newborn Mortality in Malawi: A Cross-Sectional Study. PLoS Med. 2016;13:e1002151. Medline:27755547 doi:10.1371/journal.pmed.1002151

45 Government of Malawi. Every Newborn Action Plan: an Action Plan to End Preventable Neonatal Deaths in Malawi. Malawi: Government of Malawi, 2015.

46 Government of the Republic of Malawi. National Health Policy: Towards Universal Health Coverage. Lilongwe, Malawi: Ministry of Health and Population, Government of Malawi, 2018 March, 2018. Report.

47 Government of the Republic of Malawi. Health Sector Strategic Plan II 2017-2022. Malawi: 2017.

48 Kanyangarara M, Munos MK, Walker N. Quality of antenatal care service provision in health facilities across sub–Saharan Africa: Evidence from nationally representative health facility assessments. J Glob Health. 2017;7:021101. Medline:29163936 doi:10.7189/jogh.07.021101

49 Kanyangarara M, Walker N, Boerma T. Gaps in the implementation of antenatal syphilis detection and treatment in health facilities across sub-Saharan Africa. PLoS One. 2018;13:e0198622. Medline:29856849 doi:10.1371/journal.pone.0198622

50 Nguhiu PK, Barasa EW, Chuma J. Determining the effective coverage of maternal and child health services in Kenya, using demographic and health survey data sets: tracking progress towards universal health coverage. Trop Med Int Health. 2017;22:442-53. Medline:28094465 doi:10.1111/tmi.12841

51 Hodgins S, D'Agostino A. The quality-coverage gap in antenatal care: toward better measurement of effective coverage. Glob Health Sci Pract. 2014;2:173-81. Medline:25276575 doi:10.9745/GHSP-D-13-00176

52 USAID. Malawi: Nutrition Profile. Washington DC: USAID, 2018 February 2018. Report.

53 Khan AI, Kabir I, Eneroth H, El Arifeen S, Ekstrom EC, Frongillo EA, et al. Effect of a randomised exclusive breastfeeding counselling intervention nested into the MINIMat prenatal nutrition trial in Bangladesh. Acta Paediatrica. 2017;106:49-54. Medline:27659772 doi:10.1111/apa.13601

54 Leslie HH, Hirschhorn LR, Marchant T, Doubova SV, Gureje O, Kruk ME. Health systems thinking: A new generation of research to improve healthcare quality. PLoS Med. 2018;15:e1002682. Medline:30376581 doi:10.1371/journal.pmed.1002682

55 Do M, Micah A, Brondi L, Campbell H, Marchant T, Eisele T, et al. Linking household and facility data for better coverage measures in reproductive, maternal, newborn, and child health care: systematic review. J Glob Health. 2016;6:020501. Medline:27606060 doi:10.7189/jogh.06.020501

56 Health Data Collaborative. Health Data Collaborative Progress Report 2016-2017. Health Data Collaborative, 2017 May 2017. Report No.: 1.

57 da Silva Lopes K, Ota E, Shakya P, Dagvadorj A, Balogun OO, Pena-Rosas JP, et al. Effects of nutrition interventions during pregnancy on low birth weight: an overview of systematic reviews. BMJ Glob Health. 2017;2:e000389. Medline:29018583 doi:10.1136/bmjgh-2017-000389

Section 3

Determinants of coverage

Strong community-based health systems and national governance predict improvement in coverage of oral rehydration solution (ORS): a multilevel longitudinal model

Althea Andrus[1], Robert Cohen[2], Liliana Carvajal[3], Shams El Arifeen[4], William Weiss[5,6]

[1] Alutiiq, US Department of State contractor, Washington, DC, USA

[2] CAMRIS International, Inc., USAID contractor, Bethesda, Maryland, USA

[3] UNICEF, New York, New York, USA

[4] icddr,b, Dhaka, Bangladesh

[5] Department of International Health, John Hopkins University, Baltimore, Maryland, USA

[6] Sustaining Technical and Analytic Resources (STAR) Project, Public Health Institute, USAID Contractor, Washington, DC, USA

Diarrheal disease remains a leading cause of child death globally, especially in low and middle-income countries. Use of oral rehydration solution (ORS) for treatment of diarrhea in children, a very cost-effective intervention, remains below 50% in many countries. Here we use a multi-level longitudinal model to reveal important predictors of ORS use at the national level. The findings suggest that increasing government effectiveness along with increased implementation and affordability of community-based health programs can lead to substantial increases in ORS use. Key informant interviews with national health leaders in countries that significantly improved ORS coverage support these quantitative findings.

Diarrhea remains a leading cause of death among children under five [1,2], disproportionately affecting children in low- and middle-income countries [3]. One of the most cost-effective interventions for preventing death from a case of diarrhea is to treat it with oral rehydration solution (ORS), which reduces diarrhea-specific mortality by up to 93% [4]. While there are over 50 years of evidence demonstrating the effectiveness of ORS, underutilization of ORS continues in many countries with a high burden of child mortality from diarrhea [5]. The proportion of children with an episode of diarrhea who receive ORS has increased unevenly since first introduced in the 1980s [3,6] and remains below 50% in many low- and middle-income countries (LMICs) despite new formulations or low-osmolarity ORS that make it more acceptable to children, even if not dehydrated. Scaling up the use of ORS to treat diarrhea is one of the most cost-effective ways a country can accelerate the reduction of preventable child deaths. If not done, it represents a potential missed opportunity for helping a country achieve the child mortality target of Sustainable Development Goal 3: an under-5 mortality rate of 25 per 1000 live births or lower [7]. In order to help countries scale up the use of ORS for treatment of childhood diarrhea, we seek to identify factors that are predictive of ORS use on a population level, especially those factors that are sensitive to change from investments and efforts of donors, governments and communities.

Prior studies of caretakers' management of diarrheal episodes and their care-seeking behaviors have improved understanding of what predicts ORS use in several countries. These predictors include the following: (1) community empowerment and engagement [2,3,8-13], particularly among vulnerable populations [6]; (2) the mother's level of education [14-16]; (3) access to health care [13-15]; and, (4) education among medical professionals and/or caregivers [9,10,13,17-25]. Although the studies identify predictors of ORS use across several countries, generalizable knowledge about the predictors of ORS use globally is limited, and systematic literature reviews have highlighted this gap in knowledge [3,13,14]. Bridging this gap is essential to identify the policies and population level programs that will lead to increased ORS use and fewer preventable child deaths.

This study explores the national-level predictors of ORS use globally through a quantitative model similar to the one used in the *Success factors study for reducing maternal and child mortality* [24]. That study sought to explain why some countries have reduced maternal and under-five mortality more quickly than comparable ones. The quantitative part of the *Success factors study* analyzed over 250 different health determinants and found that multi-sectoral improvements in over a dozen policy areas – including immunizations, water and sanitation, and women's education – contributed additively and synergistically to under-five mortality reduction [26-28].

We hypothesize that we can identify a set of quantitative national level predictors, measuring factors from within and outside the health system, that would enable countries to accelerate increases in ORS use at the population level (ORS coverage) if addressed alone or in combination. The value-add of this study of ORS coverage is 3-fold. First, this study includes more countries, potential predictor variables, and years of observation compared to earlier studies, and therefore the findings should be more generalizable. A second value-add is the use of a longitudinal multilevel model to compare changes in potential predictor variables with changes in ORS coverage in the same time periods. Third, this method generates estimates of the potential impact on ORS coverage from changes in identified predictor variables, aiding policymakers in setting targets.

METHODS

The analysis presented here is a secondary data analysis of publicly available data, primarily from nationally representative household surveys.

Period

We used data from 1996-2016 for two main reasons. First, the beginning of this period approximately matches the launch of the Integrated Management of Childhood Illness (IMCI) initiative in 1996 by the World Health Organization [29], with an emphasis on case management of diarrhea. Second, the period also overlaps considerably with the efforts of many countries to achieve the Millennium Development Goals. Third, some of the independent variables, most notably health financing and governance, were first reported in 1995 and 1996, respectively. The end, 2016, matches the year of the most recently available household health survey used in the analysis (such as the Demographic and Health Survey or DHS, and the Multiple-Indicator Cluster Survey or MICS [30,31]). Fourth, no studies have examined factors associated with ORS coverage on a large scale with many potential factors in this period.

Dependent variable

The dependent variable is the percent of children with diarrhea in the last two weeks who were given ORS as reported by caretakers primarily published in the DHS or MICS between 1996 and 2016 [30,31].

Independent variables

To identify the independent variables, we constructed a data set of potential predictors from the following sources: (1) predictors identified in prior studies of ORS coverage; (2) variables that were significantly associated with under-5 mortality reduction in the *Success Factors study* [26-28]; and (3) variables reflecting the timing of national child health policies. Using these criteria, we tested 34 indicators as independent variables; all downloaded from the USAID Idea database [32] (**Table 1**).

Policy variables

The WHO Global Maternal Newborn Child and Adolescent Health Policy Indicator Survey includes information about adoption of WHO recommendations for national health policies and guidelines related to maternal, newborn, child, and adolescent health [33]. We screened the survey database for child health policies that were either directly relevant to ORS or relevant to predictors

Table 1. *Results of univariable analysis**

Development Sector	Indicators
Wealth	GDP per capita in constant 2010 US$ (natural log)§
Demographics	Total fertility rate†
	Percent of population in urban areas
Governance	World Bank political stability index§
	World Bank government effectiveness index‡
	Percent of parliamentary seats held by women‡
	Percent of women with access to TV, radio, or newspaper
Water, Sanitation, Hygiene	Percent of population with improved water access†
	Percent of population with improved sanitation access
Nutrition	Percent of population with height-for-age z scores<-2 SD (stunting)
	Percent of population with a body mass index <18.5 (underweight)
	Percent of population with weight-for-height z scores<-2 SD (wasting)‡
	Percent of population with weight-for-height z scores<-3 SD (severe wasting)§
Education	Average years of education, among females age 20-24 y§
	Percent of net secondary school enrollment, among females
	Percent of net secondary school enrollment, among females lagged five-years
	Percent of net primary school enrollment, among females§
	Percent of net primary school enrollment, among females lagged ten-years§
Health System	Policy recommending management of pneumonia in the community or at home by a trained provider (yes, no)
	Percent of pregnancies with at least one antenatal care visit with a qualified medical practitioner§
	Percent of pregnancies with at least four antenatal care visits‡
	Percent of children under-five that slept under an insecticide treated net last night
	Percent of births that were in a qualified medical institution
	Percent of children under-five that had upper-respiratory symptoms and sought care from a qualified medical practitioner (care-seeking for pneumonia)†
	Percent of children under-five that have received their DPT3 immunization†
	Percent of births that were attended by a skilled birth attendant
	Percent of children under-five that had a fever and sought care from a qualified medical practitioner (care-seeking for fever)
	Number of physicians per 1000 population
	Percent of births via caesarean section‡
	Percent of newborns that were checked by a qualified medical practitioner within 48 h of birth
Health Financing	Out-of-pocket health expenditure as a percent of total health expenditure§
	Health expenditure per capita in constant 2011 international $ (natural log)§
	External health spending as a percent of government health expenditure‡
	Government health expenditure as a percent of GDP§
	Total health expenditure as a percent of GDP

GDP – gross domestic product, SD – standard deviation, DTP3 – diphtheria-tetanus-pertussis

*With the exception of 'Policy recommending management of pneumonia in the community or at home by a trained provider', all data was downloaded from the USAID Idea Database [32]. Health financing, wealth, and three of the governance indicators (stability index, governance index, and parliamentary seats) were originally sourced from the World Bank. The health system, water and sanitation, nutrition, and the remaining governance indicator (women's access to radio, TV, and news) were originally from Demographic and Health Surveys. The Education variables were originally sourced from UNESCO. The policy variable was originally sourced from WHO.

†$P < 0.1$.

‡$P < 0.05$.

§$P < 0.01$.

of ORS identified in the literature. A requirement for longitudinal analysis techniques was information about the years in which a policy was in place or not. The one policy that met this requirement was approval for childhood pneumonia to be managed with antibiotics in the community or at home by a trained provider [33]. This policy is known as community case management of pneumonia and may be a component of an integrated community case management approach (iCCM). We included this policy as a potential independent variable as a proxy for increased national interest in preventing child deaths through community programs. Because pneumonia and diarrhea are leading causes of death for children under the age of five in low and middle income countries, we believe that improvements in how pneumonia in children is being managed at the community level reflects the national interest and political will to address child mortality overall at the community level, including efforts to prevent deaths from diarrhea. For analysis purposes, the information about this policy variable was converted to a Present/Not Present dummy variable for each year from 1996- 2017 in our analytical data set.

Countries included in the analysis

All 193 United Nations member states were considered eligible for the analysis. We weighted each country equally; such that large countries did not dominate the analysis. Alternatively, to prevent the analysis from being distorted by small countries, we excluded countries where the under-5 population averaged under 150 000 children each year during the study period (with a range of 150 000 to 126 000 000 [34]). The cut-off naturally emerged in the population distribution and excludes the smallest countries that can be problematic in model estimation. We included the 103 remaining countries that had at least one population level household survey that measured ORS coverage since 1996. Of these, per the World Bank's definition in 2017, 30 were low-income countries, 43 were lower-middle income countries, and 30 were upper-middle income countries.

Data adjustments

We adjusted the data and, when necessary, transformed it to facilitate modeling. The following variables were transformed to log values to improve model fit: GDP per capita (constant 2010 USD), total health expenditure per capita (constant 2011 international $) [32]. In addition to using primary and secondary school net enrollment rates, we also used enrollment rates lagged by ten years, for primary enrollment, and five years, for secondary enrollment, to test for inclusion in the final model [32]. ORS coverage is normally distributed, and therefore, we did not need to transform the dependent variable [30,31].

Independent variables were missing data in country/y when Demographic and Health Surveys had not been conducted. In addition, because education enrollment rates were lagged, there were no data for the most recent country/y. With the exception of the policy variable for Community Case Management (CCM) for pneumonia, covariate data were not missing at random; thus, we elected not to use imputation to fill in missing data for the other variables. For countries that had data available for some years, but not all, we linearly interpolated these other variables, and when data were not available for recent years, we created a forecast using a five-year moving average of the rate of change in the indicator.

For the missing CCM data, because linear interpolation was not possible, we imputed data for four countries – Dominican Republic, Jordan, Nicaragua, and Philippines–which had no reported data. The data were imputed using linear regression with the policy variable as a dependent variable and with independent variables that had at least a 0.25 correlation with available data. These independent variables were time, percent of parliamentary seats held by women, and DPT immunization among children 12-23 months. Although imputation is a valid method to fill in missing dummy data [35] when data are missing at random, these data were not missing at random. Therefore, we interpret models using imputed data with caution and only if the results concur with models without imputed data.

Longitudinal multi-level model

Model structure

We considered the baseline model with ORS as the dependent variable and year as the independent variable. A Hausman test [36] revealed that a random-effects model was preferable because it was consistent and more efficient than a fixed-effects model (Table S1 in the **Online Supplementary Document**). Robust standard errors were used to account for mild violations of underlying assumptions. We placed no constraints on the covariance between random effects. The model had random intercepts for country and World Bank region, unstructured covariance, and no autocorrelation across time. The model also included a random coefficient for time (year of survey). The equation is:

$$y_{ij} = \beta_0 + \beta_1 \times t_j + \beta X_{ij} + \alpha_k + \mu_i + \gamma_i \times t_j + \varepsilon_{ij}$$

Where y_{ij} is the percent of children under five that had diarrhea in the last two weeks who were treated with ORS in country i in year j, X_{ij} is a matrix of independent variables in country i in year j, α_k is a random intercept for region k, μ_i is a random intercept for country i, and γ_i is a random coefficient for country i.

All analyses were conducted in STATA (StataCorp., College Station TX, USA) 14 using the *xtmixed* command [37]. The relevant Stata code was:

xtmixed ors time [variables] if year >1995 | | region: | | country: time, cov(uns)
vce(robust) mle.

Selection of covariates and parameters to include in the final model

We initially tested all 36 variables separately in the above model. We considered variables that were statistically significant at the $P < 0.10$ level in the univariable analysis as candidates for the multivariable model.

To construct the multivariable model, stepwise regression was conducted using the covariates that were found to be significant in the univariable analysis (excluding the education covariates initially, which were reported less than the other variables). After imputation and interpolation, there were 235 country-years data points for variables which were significant in the univariable analysis. We therefore restricted the multivariable analysis to these 235 country-years for model comparisons. We selected a final model based on Akaike Information Criterion, or AIC [37] because it does not penalize model complexity as much as the Bayesian Information Criterion. Once we had a final model, we ran the regression for both the restricted data set of 235 data points and all 300 available data points for those variables. For this final model of 300 data points, we then tested whether the random coefficient added predictive value (Table S2 in the **Online Supplementary Document**). We continued iteratively adding variables to the model until we could no longer find a model that had an improved AIC.

Quantifying the impact of independent variables

With our final model of the full data set, we used the coefficients and their standard errors to predict the absolute annual increase in ORS coverage based on the values of annual improvement of the independent variables at the median, 75th percentile, and 90th percentile of the sampled country-year pairs. We constructed 95% confidence intervals by multiplying 1.96 by the combined standard error for this estimate; which is as follows:

$$95\%CI = \sum_{k=1}^{n} \beta_k {}^* \mu_k \pm 1.96 {}^* \sqrt{\sum_{k=1}^{n} \sigma_k^2}$$

Where k is the nth parameter, μ represents the 50th, 75th, or 90th percentile of the nth parameter, and σ_k^2 is the standard error of β_k in the final multivariable model.

Goodness of fit

Calculating the overall goodness of fit for multilevel models can be a challenge. We utilized the traditional method of calculating R^2 using the equation

$\Sigma(\hat{y}-y_i)^2/\Sigma(yi-\bar{y})^2$, because two recent examinations of methods for calculating goodness of fit in complex models has been shown that this method has less than a 1% bias of the actual value [38,39].

Multiple analyses were conducted to assess if the model's results were impacted by missing data. After a final model was developed, we regressed the same model with a restricted data set with no missing values for education and the CCM policy. This restricted data set had 157 observations. The model was also tested with an unrestricted data set of 338 observations.

After these analyses were conducted, we applied bootstrapping methods with 100 simulations for the model with both the 235 observation data set and the full unrestricted model of 338 observations.

Key informant interviews

To better interpret the results of our analysis, we conducted open-ended data gathering with key informants. Key informants were purposively sampled. We interviewed persons identified as being knowledgeable about child health programs in countries that experienced changes in ORS coverage greater than 10 percentage points (positive or negative) between two household surveys. The countries of interest were the following: (1) Burundi – an increase in ORS coverage between 2000 and 2005 of 24 percentage points from 11% to 35%; (2) Ghana – an increase of 17 percentage points from 2006-2008 (from 29 to 46 percent) followed by a decrease of 11 points in 2008-11 period from 46 to 35 percent, and then an increase of 16 points from 2011 to 2014 (35 to 51 percent); (3) Guinea-Bissau – a decrease in ORS coverage from 2000-06 of 16 points (from 39 to 23 percent) with a later increase of 48 percentage points from 2010-14 (from 19 to 67 percent); (4) Niger – an increase of 26 percentage points from 19% in 2006 to 45% in 2012; (5) Swaziland – an increase of 19 percentage points from 2000-07 (from 66 to 85 percent), a decrease of 28 percentage points from 2007-10 (from 85 to 57 percent), followed by an increase of 27 percentage points from 2010-14 (from 57 to 84 percent); and, (6) Bangladesh – an average annual increase of five percentage points throughout the period. We identified key informants in the specific countries through contact with UNICEF country offices or personal relationships with the authors. UNICEF staff in countries and bilingual USAID colleagues translated the instrument to French or Portuguese. Main questions were followed by probing questions provided in the instrument that was emailed to informants and returned by email with their answers. These experts were asked to respond to an open-ended question about what they believed were the main reasons why ORS coverage changed in their country in the periods referenced above.

RESULTS

Changes in ORS coverage

Increases in ORS coverage between survey years are uneven. The absolute annual change in ORS coverage between surveys is normally distributed with a mean of 0.66 percentage points per year (**Figure 1**, n = 307, standard deviation = 2.9, range -12.5 to 14.5).

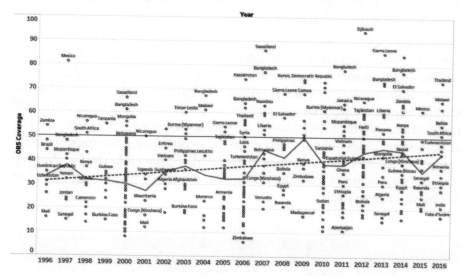

Figure 1. *Oral rehydration salt (ORS) coverage from household surveys by year, 1996-2016. The axis shows ORS coverage: the proportions of children that had diarrhea in the two-weeks prior to the household survey who received ORS in treatment of their diarrhea as reported by the child's caretaker. The x-axis shows the year in which the household survey was carried out. Each estimate of ORS coverage is (by year and country) is indicated by an open circle. The blue solid line the average ORS coverage estimates for the given year. The blue dashed line shows the linear trend in the average ORS coverage between 1996 and 2016.*

Univariable analysis

Improved ORS coverage was significantly associated with 20 of the 36 independent variables at the $P < 0.10$ level (**Table 1**; Table S3 in the **Online Supplementary Document**). These included five of twelve health system variables and four out of five health financing variables. Among the education variables, we found that primary school had a stronger correlation with ORS coverage than did secondary school. Three of the four governance variables showed a relationship with ORS coverage as did two of the four nutrition variables. Total fertility rates, GDP per capita, and access to improved water were also found to be significant in the univariable analysis.

Multivariable analysis

In addition to time, the final model included four independent variables that were selected by AIC. Backward elimination was used to try to remove excess model parameters which did not add predictive value, but all model parameters remained in the model. The independent predictor variables in the final model are the following: time, government effectiveness index, care-seeking for symptoms of pneumonia, out-of-pocket expenditures, and four or more antenatal care visits (**Table 2**; Tables S4-5 in the **Online Supplementary Document**). The OLS R^2 value was 0.90.

These results were robust to multiple sensitivity analyses. AIC preferred the same model whether we used the data set of 235 observations (Table S4 in the **Online Supplementary Document**), the more restricted data set of 157 observations with no missing values for education and CCM policy (Table S5 in the **Online Supplementary Document**), or an unrestricted data set of 300 or 338 observations in which we included all available country-years (**Table 2**). The education variables did not reach statistical significance when controlling for the other health system variables in the restricted data set. The CCM policy variable was excluded from the final model because it was not significant in the univariable analysis.

Table 2. *Regression output of final multivariable models**

	FINAL MODEL 1	FINAL MODEL 1	FINAL MODEL 2	FINAL MODEL 2	FINAL MODEL 3	FINAL MODEL 3	FINAL MODEL 4	FINAL MODEL 4
Variables	Restricted model	Bootstrap 100 reps	Unrestricted model	Bootstrap 100 reps	Restricted model	Bootstrap 100 reps	Unrestricted model	Bootstrap 100 reps
Care-seeking for pneumonia	0.152‡	0.152	0.173‡	0.173‡	0.210‡	0.210†	0.174§	0.174‡
	(0.0379)	(0.103)	(0.0174)	(0.0199)	(0.0230)	(0.00448)	(0.0895)	(0.0111)
Government effectiveness	5.804†	5.804†	4.413†	4.413§	4.323†	4.323§	5.589†	5.589†
	(2.89×10^{-7})	(0.00634)	(0.000148)	(0.0656)	(2.13×10^{-5})	(0.0506)	(0.00584)	(0.00233)
Out-of-pocket expenditures	-0.0945§	-0.0945	-0.0652‡	-0.0652	-0.0802‡	-0.0802	-0.137†	-0.137‡
	(0.0778)	(0.187)	(0.0297)	(0.278)	(0.0290)	(0.200)	(0.00510)	(0.0169)
ANC4+	0.0983§	0.0983	0.0817	0.0817				
	(0.0578)	(0.105)	(0.170)	(0.122)				
Year	0.387†	0.387†	0.388†	0.388†	0.436†	0.436†	0.525†	0.525†
	(0.00134)	(0.00265)	(0.00372)	(0.00372)	(0.00018)	(00365)	(0.00132)	(4.89×10^{-5})
Constant	21.05†	21.05†	18.45†	18.45†	20.84†	20.84†	23.18†	23.18†
	(0.00525)	(0.000231)	(0.000142)	(0.000136)	(1.43×10^{-9})	(1.20×10^{-5})	(2.19×10^{-6})	(5.39×10^{-6})
Observations	235	235	300	300	300	300	338	338
Number of regions	5	5	6	6	6	6	6	6
LogL	-859.7	-859.7	-1112	-1112	-1113	-1113	-1261	-1261

*Robust *P*-value in parentheses.
†$P < 0.01$.
‡$P < 0.05$.
*$P < 0.1$

Statistical significance remained for all variables (except ANC4) after we applied bootstrapping methods with 100 simulations for the model with 235 observations and a full unrestricted model of 338 observations (**Table 2**).

The variance of the random coefficient

The random coefficient for time (γ_i) represents the different speed at which countries improved ORS over time, after controlling for improvements in the other independent variables. For the 85 countries in the final model, γ_i was normally distributed with a mean of 0, a standard deviation of .24, and a range of -.48 to.69 The countries with the five highest values for γ_i were Bangladesh, Sierra Leone, Swaziland, Timor-Leste, and Tajikistan for whom $\gamma_i > 0.4$ (**Figure 2**). These random coefficients were consistent with faster than average progress in these countries during the duration of the study (**Figure 2**).

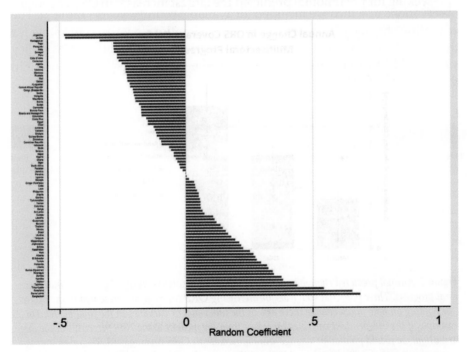

Figure 2. *Random coefficients for time by country. The random coefficients for time in the figure represent the relevant speed at which countries improved oral rehydration salt (ORS) coverage (or not) after controlling for other factors. The countries with the most rapid increases are on the right side of the figure. The countries with the five highest values (reading from left to right) are Bangladesh, Sierra Leone, Swaziland, Timor-Leste and Tajikistan. The change predicted in ORS coverage from an increase in one year, after controlling for improvements in the other independent variables.*

Potential improvements in ORS coverage given multi-sectoral progress

We used the coefficients from the final model to predict the increase in ORS that would happen in a country from changes in the independent variables in the model (Figure 3). For example, if all final model independent variables increased from the median to the 75th percentile of the distribution, we predict on average an added annual improvement in ORS coverage of 1.5% (with a range of 1%-2.1%), or a mean of 7.7% over the typical 5-year inter-survey interval. If the independent variables increased to the 90th percentile, we would predict an added annual improvement of 2.3% (with a range of 1.6%-3%), or 11.5% over a 5-year period. These predicted improvements compare favorably to the current average annual rate of increase of 0.8%, or 4.1% over a 5-year period (see **Figure 3**). In addition, improvements in maternal and child health indicators at the primary care level (four or more antenatal care visits and care-seeking for pneumonia) predicted the largest increases in ORS coverage.

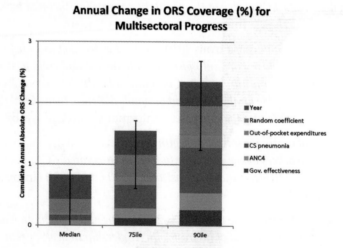

Figure 3. *Annual predicted change in oral rehydration salt (ORS) coverage by level of multi-sectoral progress. Three potential scenarios for increasing ORS coverage are presented in the figure, depending on how much change there was in the independent variables in the final model. For example, if the independent variables increased from the median to the 75th percentile of the distribution, we would predict an average annual increase in ORS coverage of 1.5%, or an average annual increase of 2.3% if increased to the 90th percentile of the distribution. This represents a substantial change of 7.7% or 11.5% or a five-year period, respectively. The figure also shows the components of the predicted increases in ORS coverage based on the independent variables in the final model. The x-axis shows increases in covariate values at median, 75th percentile, and 90th percentile levels. The y-axis shows the predicted increase in ORS coverage following increases in covariates at the three levels. Covariates include time (year), out of pocket expenditures, care-seeking for pneumonia, four or more antenatal care visits, government effectiveness, and a random coefficient.*

Key informant interviews

After contacting eight informants in six countries, we only obtained responses from two informants each in Bangladesh, Burundi, and Guinea Bissau (total of six informants). Responses from these informants supported the use of the independent variables we had included in the final model and the results. Commonly mentioned reasons across informants suggest that the following factors were salient in affecting levels of ORS use: policies and programs supporting integrated management of childhood illness (IMCI) in health facilities, health promotion in the community, and treatment of childhood illness by community health workers (community case management).

"I think that from 2000 to 2010 [period of a drop in ORS coverage] the ORS were only available for the population through health centers, which may justify the low coverage. The increase in [ORS] coverage between 2010 and 2014 could be related to the initiation of CHWs activities in some regions of the country. As a result, there was an increase in the availability of ORS as well as in the knowledge of the population regarding the need for ORS in cases of diarrhea." (Informant from Guinea-Bissau)

[Period of ORS increase from 2010-2014] *"In 2013 the so-called PIMI project started, which is mainly focused on maternal and child health interventions at community level by Community Health Workers (CHWs). These are responsible for the treatment of simple diarrhea, using Oral Rehydration Salts (ORS) for that purpose."* (Informant from Guinea-Bissau)

"Training of health personnel at health center level in IMCI and community health workers at the community level in integrated CCM [were the main reasons ORS use increased between 2000 and 2005]. (Informant from Burundi)

[Period of ORS increase from 2000-2005] *"The health promotion activities experienced a revival of interest with [leadership in health promotion that] was very active. These activities are effective when there is ownership at all levels. The central level provided impetus for implementation of these activities at the decentralized and operational level which in turn carried out sensitization at the community level. Thus, healthcare providers and communities were well aware of the benefits of ORS in treatment of childhood diarrhea and adopted the practice at scale. The fact that health personnel and caretakers of children understood the benefits and the impact of use of ORS in treatment of childhood diarrhea as well as the interest in the use of ORS for treatment childhood diarrhea was eliciting in the public health domain catalyzed the increase in coverage of ORS uptake."* (Informant from Burundi)

"The National Control of Diarrheal Diseases (CDD) program launched a nationwide ORT communication campaign in 1996 using a wide variety of communication channels to improve knowledge and awareness in the community on key rules of homecare- increased fluid, continued feeding and appropriate care-seeking during diarrhea... These campaigns reached a wide variety of community members and stakeholders including health providers and created an environment conducive to behavior change to adopt ORT and ORS as the tool for diarrhea management. The effect of these communication and promotional activities continued during the following years and created an increasingly sustained behavior of the community in using ORT and ORS during a diarrhea episode." (Informant from Bangladesh).

"The CDD program did a nationwide campaign in 1996 and continued following years to increase knowledge and awareness among the community people regarding oral rehydration therapy (ORT), continued feeding, proper care seeking for diarrhea. This multi- dimensional approach for increasing awareness among the community people, health care providers and other stakeholders was very successful and brought positive changes in attitude and practice of the population regarding treatment and care seeking behavior of diarrheal disease.... After closing of CDD program in 1998 Govt. of Bangladesh adopted WHO and UNICEF recommended Integrated Management of Childhood Illnesses (IMCI) as integrated strategy to fight child illness. Management of diarrhea was incorporated in that strategy. This helped significantly in institutionalization of ORS as a tool for management of diarrhea." (Informant from Bangladesh)

One variable, stocks of ORS, was mentioned by several informants as a critical reason for increases and decreases in ORS use. However, this variable was not included in the final model because we could not identify publicly available data on ORS stocks for each year of the analysis and across most of the countries.

[Period of ORS increase from 2000-2005] *"Health workers monitored the ORS stock levels closely and regularly made requisitions when the minimum stock level was attained on time to avoid stock-outs. Thus, ORS was available in health facilities on a regular basis and used to treat childhood diarrhea without any issues with stock-outs."* (Informant from Burundi)

[Period of ORS increase from 2010-2014] *"...Therefore, the availability of ORS is guaranteed by UNICEF and distributed in five out of the eleven sanitary regions in the country. Same distribution is carried out at health centers level."* (Informant from Guinea Bissau)

"Later the govt. ...did an agreement with SMC (Social Marketing Company), the largest social marketing company of Bangladesh. SMC started to

produce ORS and marketed it throughout the country branded as ORSa-line. ORS became available at the health facilities, local markets as well as to the depot holders. Depot holders were female community members, who were trained, used to collect ORS packets from the SMC at a subsidized price and distributed those to the community at market price. Hence ORS became available and accessible throughout the country." (Informant from Bangladesh)

"In 2003, the WHO recommended a low osmolality ORS (ORSaline–N) for childhood diarrhea management given its superior efficacy. Adopting the recommendation, SMC switched to ORSaline–N and with the support of USAID built a manufacturing plant for mass production and national distribution ORS. Now, all public and private sector companies produce low osmolality ORS. The easy-to-use ORS packets available at a cheaper price played a key role in increasing ORS use in Bangladesh." (Informant from Bangladesh)

DISCUSSION

Despite substantial progress in preventing child deaths since 1990, diarrhea was responsible for approximately 0.5 million such deaths globally in 2015 [1]. Among 129 surveys in low and middle-income countries since 2010 that assessed ORS use, the mean estimate of ORS use to treat children with diarrhea was 42% (with a range of 11%-94%). Since ORS is one of the most cost-effective interventions for preventing child deaths from diarrhea [40] and is a recommended intervention by Unicef and WHO [41] and under IMCI, this finding implies that there are ample missed opportunities to prevent many child deaths. This study suggests that a combination of strengthening the government, carrying out maternal and child health programs at the community level, and making these programs more affordable, can accelerate the use of ORS to treat childhood diarrhea on a population level. This is indicated by the associations identified in the study between increased ORS use, increased government effectiveness index, reduced out of pocket expenditures, and the increase in population coverage of the two maternal and child health interventions in the model: (1) four or more antenatal care visits and (2) care-seeking for pneumonia. There is some additional supportive evidence for these findings. From the time IMCI was introduced in the late to mid-1990s, at least until the mid-late 2000s when integrated community case management became a new focus, the program to control diarrheal diseases became more narrow, focusing on training first-level health facility workers, and losing much of the emphasis on diarrhea management in the home or availability of affordable ORS in the community (Fontaine O., personal communication) [42].

The Success Factors study found that health system improvements explained approximately half of global under-five mortality reduction from 1990-2010, while the improvements outside the health system–such as governance, water and sanitation, GDP per capita, women's empowerment and education–explained the remainder [26,27]. Our study further supports that governance plays a vital role in improving child health, which is unsurprising considering governance is one of the six health system building blocks identified by WHO [43]. Political stability not making it into the final model only because government effectiveness and political stability are highly correlated. There is a strong association with ORS coverage and the political stability index in the univariable and multivariable analyses. Governance improvement is difficult to achieve, but efforts toward this end may result in improvements in child health when combined with other efforts. National governments and donors can interpret these findings to imply that accelerating the scale-up of key child health interventions, such as ORS, requires working at all levels of the health system from policies to community level programming. There also may be added synergies from increased financing (including decreased out-of-pocket expenditures) and improved government effectiveness [44].

Of the five health financing variables we tested, only out-of-pocket health expenditures remained significant in a multivariable model, and only weakly so. This finding implies a cautious interpretation that all of the health financing variables, such as total health spending in the country, affect ORS use by affecting access. Access to care was already adequately controlled for by the other variables in our model such as antenatal care and care-seeking for pneumonia. Financial limitations are, however, a potentially severe bottleneck in health care access, and our findings do not discount their importance.

The key informant interviews (KIIs) that we conducted further supports our interpretation. Representatives from Guinea-Bissau and Burundi confirmed the importance of effective government in improved ORS use. The respondents from Burundi stated that "ownership at all levels of the health system," contributed to periods of expanded ORS use. In Guinea-Bissau, the respondents suggested that the reason ORS increased sharply from 2010-2014 was due to the deployment of community health workers in 2013 as part of a specific child health project in the country, and a decrease in political crises which would allow for more effective government index values. Informants from Bangladesh stressed the importance of national policies in increasing ORS use.

The significant spread of the random coefficient (**Figure 2**) and the contribution of time to improvements in ORS coverage (**Figure 3**) imply that, after controlling for the other factors in the model, approximately one-quarter of ORS improvements can be attributed to activities that were unmeasured and/or unique to the individual countries. The KIIs reflect such activities. A country seeking to reduce child diarrhea mortality dramatically–as Bangladesh achieved–could implement diarrhea-specific programming to accelerate progress.

Limitations

Due to the limitations of this analysis, some caution is warranted. First, health indicators were only available for 235 data points. Cross-country regressions are known to be sensitive to non-random data availability, and while the statistical significance of several variables – such as government effectiveness and care-seeking pneumonia – were consistent; other variables were less consistently associated with improvements [43]. Second, these indicators are presumably proxies for health system strengthening; it is unlikely that increasing care-seeking for pneumonia will cause ORS coverage to also increase. Furthermore, national estimates do not always proxy well for subnational variation.

While the robustness of our findings, and the relatively high value for R^2, increases our confidence–whether we included the full or restricted data set and after bootstrapping standard errors–we still may not have had sufficient statistical power to detect relationships for some of the other variables or they may be critical in omitted countries. Other variables that may be drivers of ORS coverage, such as community health worker density or severity of the diarrhea cases were not available and should be included in future analyses. We might expect ORS use to be higher where there are more trained health workers and in cases where the diarrhea was severe. Also, we were unable to include in our analysis information about the availability or stock of ORS, although key informants suggest that this would have been important to include in our model. Finally, while the longitudinal structure of our model strengthens our ability to make a causal inference, this remains a non-random retrospective analysis. Importantly, this analysis did not assess changes in zinc coverage, which has been shown to significantly impact morbidity when used in combination with ORS for treatment of diarrhea but often has significantly lower coverage [20]. Countdown to 2030 recommends integrating zinc with ORS in child health programming [44].

The variables dropped from the multivariable analysis are equally as important to note. GDP per capita, total fertility rates, clean water access, and maternal education all associated strongly with ORS coverage in univariable analyses (and maternal education is associated with ORS use in prior literature). However, these associations were not significant when controlling for other predictors of ORS coverage. While these indicators remain crucial for overall child mortality reduction, these findings imply that ORS coverage can be improved significantly even at low poverty or high fertility rates, probably through health system interventions (ie, deployment of community health workers, or demand generation) and improved governance.

Information provided by key informants was included to help the authors and readers interpret the finding of the analysis. The key informants were purposively selected from countries with relatively large changes in ORS coverage and therefore do not represent the full spectrum of countries in the study.

CONCLUSION

Increasing ORS coverage can help prevent many child deaths between now and 2030, a target of Sustainable Development Goal 3. Much room for improving the treatment of childhood diarrhea with ORS remains, however. One path to increasing ORS coverage appears to lie mainly in reinvigorating known approaches to improving maternal and child health (demand generation, deployment of human resources and health promotion activities at the community level), and improved governance. Effective and affordable community health programs can play a vital role in improving the coverage of cost-effective child health services.

Acknowledgments: The authors would like to acknowledge the Countdown to 2030 members, Neal Brandes, Patricia Jodrey and Olivier Fontaine for their comments and recommendations for improving this manuscript. We also give special acknowledgement to the key informants who provided better understanding of our findings.

Disclaimer: Note that the authors' views expressed in this publication do not necessarily reflect the views of the United States Government.

Ethics approval: The Johns Hopkins School of Public Health Institutional Review Board determined that this project does not meet the definition of "human subjects research" as defined by DHHS regulations 45 CFR 46.102, and does not require IRB oversight. The project involved secondary analysis of an existing, publicly available de-identified data set and conducted interviews with key informants about changes in coverage of diarrhea treatment with oral rehydration solution in low- and middle-income countries. No personal or private information was collected.

Funding: Some authors received salary support to develop the manuscript: AD received salary from the Public Health Institute (a US Agency for International Development contractor); RC received salary from CAMRIS International, Inc. (a US Agency for International Development contractor); and, WW received salary from The John Hopkins University (under an Inter-Agency Personnel Agreement between the university and the US Agency for International Development) and from the Public Health Institute (a US Agency for International Development contractor).

Authorship contributions: AA wrote most of the original draft of the manuscript, compiled the data for analysis, and performed some analysis. RC performed most of the quantitative analysis including data tables, wrote portions of the methods, results, and discussion sections, provided feedback and edits to drafts of the manuscript. LC provided key advice on the elements and direction of the analysis, identified and arranged for interviews with key informants and wrote sections of the methods, provided feedback and edits to drafts of the manuscript. SA provided key advice on the elements and direction of the analysis and provided feedback and edits to drafts of the manuscript. WW developed the concept for the manuscript and the outline of the manuscript, provided overall direction for the quantitative and qualitative analysis approach, analyzed the qualitative data, and wrote the original drafts of the discussion and conclusions.

Competing interests: The authors completed the Unified Competing Interest form at www.icmje.org/coi_disclosure.pdf (available upon request from the corresponding author), and declare no conflicts of interest.

Additional material
Online Supplementary Document

References

1   Liu L, Oza S, Hogan D, Chu Y, Perin J, Zhu J, et al. Global, regional, and national causes of under-5 mortality in 2000-15: an updated systematic analysis with implications for the Sustainable Development goals. Lancet. 2016;388:3027-35. Medline:27839855 doi:10.1016/S0140-6736(16)31593-8

2   Ghimire PR, Agho KE, Renzaho AMN, Dibley M, Raynes-Greenow C. Association between health service use and diarrhoea management approach among caregivers of under-five children in Nepal. PLoS One. 2018;13:e0191988. Medline:29494611 doi:10.1371/journal.pone.0191988

3   Lenters LM, Das JK, Bhutta ZA. Systematic review of strategies to increase use of oral rehydration solution at the household level. BMC Public Health. 2013;13(Suppl 3):S28. Medline:24564428 doi:10.1186/1471-2458-13-S3-S28

4   Munos MK, Walker CLF, Black RE. The effect of oral rehydration solution and recommended home fluids on diarrhoea mortality. Int J Epidemiol. 2010;39(Suppl 1):i75-87. Medline:20348131 doi:10.1093/ije/dyq025

5   Nalin DR. Cash, Richard A. 50 years of oral rehydration therapy: the solution is still simple. Lancet. 2018;392:536-8. Medline:30152375 doi:10.1016/S0140-6736(18)31488-0

6   Forsberg BC, Petzold M, Tomson G, Allebeck P. Diarrhoea case management in low- and middle-income countries–an unfinished agenda. Bull World Health Organ. 2007;85:42-8. Medline:17242757 doi:10.2471/BLT.06.030866

7   United Nations Progress towards the Sustainable Development Goals. 2017. Available: https://sustainabledevelopment.un.org/sdg3. Accessed: 30 June 2018.

8   Bachrach LR, Gardner JM. Caregiver knowledge, attitudes, and practices regarding childhood diarrhea and dehydration in Kingston, Jamaica. Rev Panam Salud Publica. 2002;12:37-44. Medline:12202023 doi:10.1590/S1020-49892002000700006

9   Wilson SE, Ouedraogo CT, Prince L, Ouedraogo A, Hess SY, Rouamba N, et al. Caregiver recognition of childhood diarrhea, care seeking behaviors and home treatment practices in rural Burkina Faso: A Cross-Sectional Survey. PLoS One. 2012;7:e33273. Medline:22428006 doi:10.1371/journal.pone.0033273

10   Olson CK, Blum LS, Patel KN, Oria P, Feikin DR, Laserson KF, et al. Community case management of childhood diarrhea in a setting with declining use of oral rehydration therapy: Findings from cross-sectional studies among primary household caregivers, Kenya, 2007. Am J Trop Med Hyg. 2011;85:1134-40. Medline:22144458 doi:10.4269/ajtmh.2011.11-0178

11   Charyeva Z, Cannon M, Oguntunde O, Garba AM, Sambisa W, Bassi AP, et al. Reducing the burden of diarrhea among children under five years old: lessons learned from oral rehydration therapy corner program implementation in Northern Nigeria. J Health Popul Nutr. 2015;34:4-8. Medline:26825053 doi:10.1186/s41043-015-0005-1

12   Othero DM, Otengah PA, Kaseje DO, Orago AS, Groenewegen T. Home management of diarrhea among underfives in a rural community in Kenya: Household Perceptions and practices. East Afr J Public Health. 2008;5:142-6. Medline:19374313

13   Hill Z, Kendall C, Arthur P, Kirkwood B, Adjei E. Recognizing childhood illnesses and their traditional explanations: exploring options for care-seeking interventions in the context of the IMCI strategy in rural Ghana. Trop Med Int Health. 2003;8:668-76. Medline:12828551 doi:10.1046/j.1365-3156.2003.01058.x

14   Stallings R. Child Morbidity and treatment patterns. Calverton, Maryland: support provided by USAID; 2004 p. 7–66. (DHS Comparative Reports). Report No.: 8. Available: https://dhsprogram.com/pubs/pdf/CR8/CR8.pdf. Accessed: 5 March 2018.

15   Geldsetzer P, Williams TC, Kirolos A, Mitchell S, Ratcliffe LA, Kohli-Lynch MK, et al. The recognition of and care seeking behaviour for childhood illness in developing countries: A systematic review. PLoS One. 2014;9:e93427. Medline:24718483 doi:10.1371/journal.pone.0093427

16   Coreil J, Genece E. Adoption of oral rehydration therapy among Haitian mothers. Soc Sci Med. 1988;27:87-96. Medline:3212508 doi:10.1016/0277-9536(88)90166-9

17   Reis EC, Goepp JG, Katz S, Santosham M. Barriers to use of oral rehydration therapy. Pediatrics. 1994;93:708-11. Medline:8165066

18   Costa AD, da Silva GAP. Oral rehydration therapy in emergency departments. J Pediatr (Rio J). 2011;87:175-9. Medline:21503384 doi:10.2223/JPED.2066

19   Baqui AH, Black RE, El Arifeen S, Yunus M, Zaman K, Begum N, et al. Zinc therapy for diarrhoea increased the use of oral rehydration therapy and reduced the use of antibiotics in Bangladeshi Children. J Health Popul Nutr. 2004;22:440-2. Medline:15663177

20   Blum LS, Oria PA, Olson CK, Breiman RF, Ram PK. Examining the use of oral rehydration salts and other oral rehydration therapy for childhood diarrhea in Kenya. Am J Trop Med Hyg. 2011;85:1126-33. Medline:22144457 doi:10.4269/ajtmh.2011.11-0171

21   Digre N, Moodley M, Digre P, Simpson E, Cali S, Lartey B. Caregiver perceptions and utilization of oral rehydration solution and other treatments for diarrhea among young children in Burkina Faso. J Glob Health. 2016;6:020407. Medline:27699000 doi:10.7189/jogh.06.020407

22   Cogswell ME, Oni GA, Stallings RY, Brown KH. Sociodemographic and clinical factors affecting recognition of childhood diarrhea by mothers in Kwara State, Nigeria. Soc Sci Med. 1991;33:1209-16. Medline:1767291 doi:10.1016/0277-9536(91)90237-7

23   Widarsa KT, Muninjaya AG. Factors associated with the use of oral rehydration solution among mothers in West Lombok, Indonesia. J Diarrhoeal Dis Res. 1994;12:261-4. Medline:7751566

24   Jain H, Bamnawat S. Knowledge and attitude towards oral rehydration therapy among mothers of under-five children of South Rajasthan, India. Int J Contemp Pediat. 2016;3:394-7. doi:10.18203/2349-3291.ijcp20161021

25   Desta BK, Assimamaw NT, Ashenaf TD. Knowledge, practice, and associated factors of home-based management of diarrhea among caregivers of children attending under-five clinic in Fagita Lekoma District, Awi Zone, Amhara Regional State, Northwest Ethiopia, 2016. Hindawi. Nurs Res Pract. 2017;2017:8084548. Medline:28912970 doi:10.1155/2017/8084548

26 Kuruvilla S, Schweitzer J, Bishai D, Chowdhury S, Caramani D, Frost L, et al. Success factors for reducing maternal and child mortality. Bull World Health Organ. 2014;92:533-44B. Medline:25110379 doi:10.2471/BLT.14.138131

27 Bishai DM, Cohen R, Alfonso YN, Taghreed A, Kuruvilla S, Schweitzer J. Factors contributing to maternal and child mortality reductions in 146 low- and middle-income countries between 1990 and 2010. PLoS One. 2016;11:e0144908. Medline:26783759 doi:10.1371/journal.pone.0144908

28 Cohen RL, Murray J, Jack S, Arscott-Mills S, Verardi V. Impact of multisectoral health determinants on child mortality 1980-2010: An analysis by country baseline mortality. PLoS One. 2017;12:e0188762. Medline:29211765 doi:10.1371/journal.pone.0188762

29 Costello A, Daglish S. Towards a grand convergence for child survival and health. Geneva: WHO; 2016.

30 International ICF. Demographic and health surveys. Calverton, Maryland: ICF International; 1996 2017. Available: https://www.statcompiler.com/en/. Accessed: 21 June 2018.

31 International ICF. Multiple indicator cluster surveys. Calverton, Maryland: ICF International; 1996 2017. Available: https://www.statcompiler.com/en/. Accessed: 21 June 2018.

32 USAID. International Data & Economic Analysis (IDEA). Available: https://idea.usaid.gov/about.html#tab-about. Accessed: 7 May 2017.

33 WHO Department of Maternal, Newborn, child and adolescent health. Global Maternal Newborn Child and Adolescent Health Policy Indicator Survey. 2009 2016.

34 United Nations Population Division. World population prospects 2017. New York, New York: United Nations; Available: https://esa.un.org/unpd/wpp/DataSources/. Accessed: 21 June 2018.

35 Allison PD. Imputation of categorical variables with PROC MI. Focus Session Paper 113-30 presented at: 30th Meeting of SAS User Group International; 2005; Philadelphia, PA.

36 Hausman J. Specification Tests in Econometrics. Econometrica. 1978;46:1251-71. doi:10.2307/1913827

37 Akaike H. Maximum likelihood identification of Gaussian autoregressive moving average models. Biometrika. 1973;60:255-65. doi:10.1093/biomet/60.2.255

38 LaHuis DM, Hartman MJ, Hakoyama S, Clark PC. Explained Variance measures for multilevel models. Organ Res Methods. 2014;17:2014. doi:10.1177/1094428114541701

39 Nakagawa S, Schielzeth H. A general and simple method for obtaining R^2 from generalized linear mixed-effects models. Methods Ecol Evol. 2013;4:133-42. doi:10.1111/j.2041-210x.2012.00261.x

40 Health Statistics and Information Systems: Disease Burden and Mortality Estimates. Geneva: WHO; 2018.

41 Keusch GT, Walker CF, Das JK, Horton S, Habte D. Diarrheal diseases. In: Reproductive, maternal, newborn, and child health. 3rd ed. Washington, DC: The World Bank; 2016.

42 Black R, Fontaine O, Lamberti L, Bhan M, Huicho L, El Arifeen S, et al. Drivers of the reduction in childhood diarrhea mortality 1980-2015 and interventions to eliminate preventable diarrhea deaths by 2030. J Glob Health. 2019;9:020801. Medline:31673345 doi:10.7189/jogh.09.020801

43 WHO's Framework for Action. Everybody's business: strengthening health systems to improve health outcomes. Geneva, Switzerland: World Health Organization; 2007. Available: https://apps.who.int/iris/handle/10665/43918. Accessed: 8 June 2018.

44 Boerma T, Requejo J, Victora C. Tracking progress towards universal coverage for reproductive, newborn and child health. Washington, DC: United Nations Children's Fund and the World Health Organization; 2017. Report No.: The 2017 Report. Available: http://countdown2030.org/pdf/Countdown-2030-complete-with-profiles.pdf. Accessed: 8 June 2018.

Appendix 1.

Links to online supplementary documents.

Online supplementary materials for chapter:

Timing and number of antenatal care contacts in low and middle-income countries: Analysis in the Countdown to 2030 priority countries.

http://jogh.org/documents/issue202001/jogh-10-010502-s001.pdf

Online supplementary materials for chapter:

Strong community-based health systems and national governance predict improvement in coverage of oral rehydration solution (ORS): a multilevel longitudinal model.

http://jogh.org/documents/issue202001/jogh-10-010503-s001.zip

Online supplementary materials for chapter:

Discordance in postnatal care between mothers and newborns: Measurement artifact or missed opportunity?

http://jogh.org/documents/issue202001/jogh-10-010505-s001.pdf

Online supplementary materials for chapter:

Variance estimation for effective coverage measures: A simulation study.

http://jogh.org/documents/issue202001/jogh-10-010506-s001.zip

Online supplementary materials for chapter:

Basic maternal health care coverage among adolescents in 22 sub-Saharan African countries with high adolescent birth rate

http://jogh.org/documents/issue202001/jogh-10-020401-s001.pdf